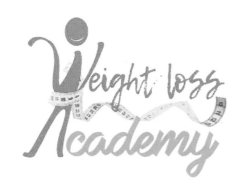

Mediterranean Diet Cookbook For Beginners 2021

And

The Ultimate Keto Guide for Beginners after 50

|2 BOOKS IN 1|

120+ Quick & Easy Delicious Recipes to Build Habits of Health | Change your Eating Lifestyle with 16 Weeks Smart Meal Plan!

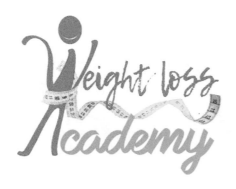

Mediterranean Diet Cookbook For Beginners 2021

70+ Fresh and Foolproof Recipes with 21-Day Meal Plan for a Healthy Lifestyle

Table Of Contents

BOOK: 1 Mediterranean Diet Cookbook

Introduction 1

What is Mediterranean Diet?............................... 2

What are the benefits of Mediterranean Diet? 4

How to get started? 6

21 Days Meal Plan.. 8

MEDITERRANEAN DIET BREAKFAST RECIPES 10

Spinach and Artichoke Frittata.................................11

Hearty Breakfast Fruit Salad.....................................12

Shakshuka 14

Caprese Avocado Toast...15

Spinach Feta Breakfast Wraps..................................16

Easy Homemade Muesli..17

Kale and Goat Cheese Frittata Cups 18

Easy, Fluffy Lemon Ricotta Pancakes 19

Smashed Egg Toasts with Herby Lemon Yogurt 20

Mediterranean Breakfast Pitas.................................21

Crispy White Beans with Greens and Poached Egg 22

Breakfast Grain Salad with Blueberries, Hazelnuts &
Lemon 23

Eggs with Summer Tomatoes, Zucchini, and Bell
Peppers 24

Avocado and Egg Breakfast Pizza 25

Mediterranean Breakfast Sandwich 26

Breakfast Hash with Brussels Sprouts and Sweet
Potatoes..27

Mediterranean Keto Low Carb Egg Muffins with
Ham 29

Mediterranean Diet Lunch Recipes 30

Mediterranean Chickpea Quinoa Bowl......................31

Tomato Salad with Grilled Halloumi and Herbs 32

Harissa Chickpea Stew with Eggplant and Millet........33

Five-Minute Heirloom Tomato Toast.........................35

Eggplant and Herb Flatbread....................................36

5-Minute Mediterranean Couscous with Tuna and
Pepperoncini 37

Pesto Quinoa Bowls With Roasted Veggies and
Labneh 38

Greek Yogurt Chicken Salad Stuffed Peppers.............39

15-Minute Mezze Plate with Toasted Za ' atar Pita
Bread 40

Greek Lemon Chicken Skewers with Tzatziki Sauce....41

This Eggplant Pizza is Low-Carb, Gluten-Free and
Ready in Under An Hour 42

Wild Alaska Salmon and Smashed Cucumber Grain
Bowls 43

Harissa Potato Salad 44

Greek Lemon Chicken Soup 45

Mediterranean Bento Lunch 46

Greek Meatball Mezze Bowls....................................47

Mediterranean Chicken with Orzo Salad 48

MEDITERRANEAN DIET DINNER RECIPES 49

Mediterranean Portobello Mushroom Pizzas with
Arugula Salad 50

Slow-Cooker Mediterranean Quinoa with Arugula 51

Walnut-Rosemary Crusted Salmon 52

Mediterranean Stuffed Chicken Breasts....................53

Charred Shrimp & Pesto Buddha Bowls....................54

Sheet-Pan Salmon with Sweet Potatoes & Broccoli ...55

Greek Cauliflower Rice Bowls with Grilled Chicken....56

Prosciutto Pizza with Corn & Arugula.......................57

Vegan Mediterranean Lentil Soup.............................58

BBQ Shrimp with Garlicky Kale & Parmesan-Herb
Couscous..59

Green Shakshuka with Spinach, Chard & Feta 60

One-Skillet Salmon with Fennel & Sun-Dried Tomato
Couscous...61

Chicken & Spinach Skillet Pasta with Lemon &
Parmesan..62

Baked chicken and Ricotta Meatballs.......................63

Chickpea Vegetable Coconut Curry 65

Broccoli Rabe and Burrata with Lemon 66

Tomato Poached Cod with Special Herbs 67

Chickpea Shawarma Salad 68

Mediterranean Diet Snacks Recipes 70

Minute Mediterranean Chickpea Salad 71

Lemon Herb Mediterranean Pasta Salad 72

Hummus 73

Mini Greek Pita Pizzas...74

Healthy Avocado Cilantro White Bean Dip 75

Homemade Granola Bars Recipe (Gluten-Free,
Vegan, Dairy-Free)...76

Charcuterie Bistro Lunch Box 77

Hummus, Feta & Bell Pepper Cracker 78

Tomato-Basil Skewers 79

Marinated Olives & Feta...80

Garlic Hummus...81

Clementine & Pistachio Ricotta................................82

Ricotta & Yogurt Parfait...83

Mediterranean Picnic Snacks 84

Crock Pot Chunky Monkey Paleo Trail Mix Recipe 85

Savory Feta Spinach and Sweet Red Pepper Muffins .86

Smoked Salmon, Avocado and Cucumber Bites........87

Conclusion 88

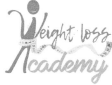

BOOK 2: Keto diet After 50 for Beginners

Introduction 92
    Is the Keto Diet Healthy for People Over 50?............93
    The Keto Mistakes Everyone Makes 96
How to Get into Ketosis 99
    Ketogenic Vs Low Carb.................................99
    What Is Ketosis? 99
    Foods Allowed in Keto Diet................................101
    Foods authorized in moderate quantities..............104
Benefit of Keto Diet for People Over 50 105
    Benefits Ketogenic Diet.............................105
    Risk of a Ketogenic Diet 107
Keto Grocery List 110
28 Days Meal Plan............................... 115
Breakfast 117
    Antipasti Skewers 118
    Kale, Edamame and Tofu Curry 119
    Chocolate Cupcakes with Matcha Icing 120
    Sesame Chicken Salad 121
    Jalapeno Poppers 122
    BLT Party Bites.......................................123
    Strawberries and Cream Smoothie.....................124
    Preparation Time: 5 minutes.........................124
    Cauli Flitters 125
    Bacon Wrapped Chicken................................126
    No-Bake Keto Power Bars 127
Lunch 128
    Buttered Cod..129
    Salmon with Red Curry Sauce 130
    Salmon Teriyaki 131
    Pesto Shrimp with Zucchini Noodles 132
    Crab Cakes..133
    Tuna Salad..135
    Keto Frosty...136
    Keto Shake 137
    Keto Fat Bombs 138
    Avocado Ice Pops......................................139

Dinner..140
    Beef-Stuffed Mushrooms...............................141
    Rib Roast...142
    Beef Stir Fry...143
    Sweet & Sour Pork.....................................144
    Grilled Pork with Salsa 145
    Garlic Pork Loin 146
    Chicken Pesto...147
    Garlic Parmesan Chicken Wings 148
    Crispy Baked Shrimp...................................149
    Herbed Mediterranean Fish Fillet 150
Vegetables..151
    Tomato and broccoli soup 152
    Bok Choy Stir Fry with Fried Bacon Slices 153
    Broccoli-cauliflower stew.............................154
    Creamy Avocado Soup...................................155
    Bok choy mushroom soup 156
    Tasty Radish Soup.....................................157
    Fried garlicy bacon and bok choy broth................158
    Nutritional Mustard Greens and Spinach Soup.......159
    Hash Browns with Radish 160
    Baked Radishes 161
Poultry...162
    Pancakes..163
    Cheese Roll-Ups 164
    Scrambled Eggs with Spinach and Cheese 165
    Egg Wraps...166
    Chaffles with Poached Eggs 167
    Chaffle with Scrambled Eggs 168
    Sheet Pan Eggs with Mushrooms and Spinach........169
    Sandwich..170
    Scrambled Eggs with Basil and Butter 171
    Bacon, and Eggs 172
    Boiled Eggs 173
Conclusion 175

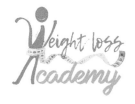

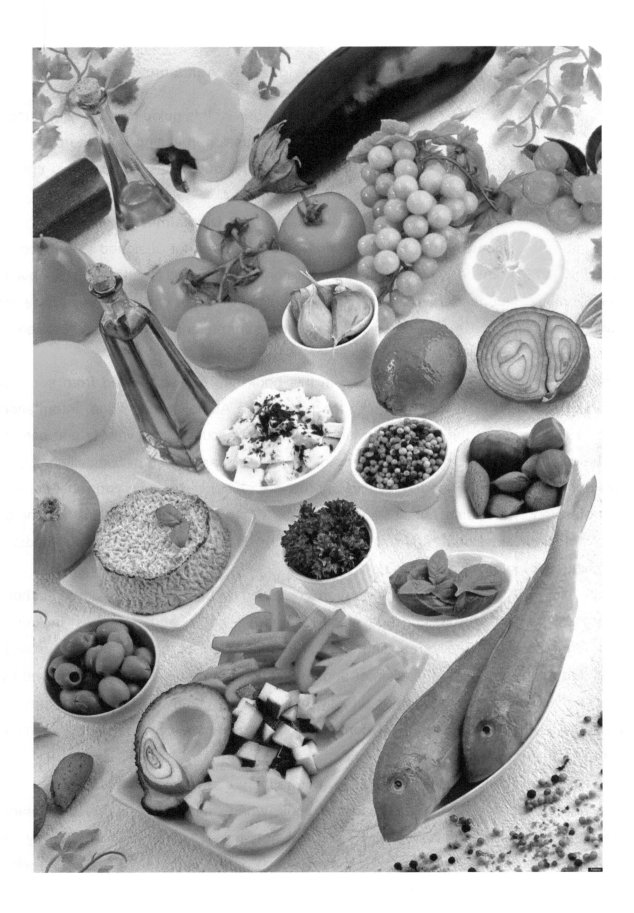

Introduction

If you have ever noticed the health of people today, especially teenagers, and the food items that fill their platter, you may not take much time to find the type of health they possess. Their little, partial or full obesity may find its reason in pizza, white bread, refined sugar, processed food they eat which has many preservatives. The taste buds seem to reign supreme in the kingdom of food.

But the analysis and research on processed food items like frozen food, white bread and carbonated drinks, has brought startling facts forward. It has surfaced in some of the research findings that huge and habitual consumption of these items can tax the body. Its over consumption can result in high production of insulin. This can cause the risk of diabetes, obesity and coronary malfunction.

The reality of animal fat is not much different. The saturated fats in these food items can have adverse effect on our body. It causes accumulation of extra fats in our body and disturbs our body mass index. The saturated fat in animal products milk and butter increases bad cholesterol-LDL. In short, it can harm coronary health

In this technologically advanced when with little efforts we can accomplish our tasks. Physical activities are negligible. Poor health comfortably steps in. It becomes essential to switch to healthier diet which fulfils the nutrition need of our body and at the same time keeps us filled. There is much information on nutrition filled diet. However, it is difficult to make a choice.

Nonetheless when we have visible effects of centuries, over generations of people, we can trust it to some extent. A nutrition analysis can help make our trust stay longer in it. This is true about Mediterranean diet. A food pattern which brims with whole grains, plant based diet has olive oil as a source of fats and other items which provide calories essential for our body. This diet has no space for processed food is loaded with sugar or artificial sweeteners. As a result the low amount of fats keeps the heart healthy, provides both the essential nutrients and agility. Give it a start, I feel you won't look back. You will rather leap into a healthy future.

"Wish you a healthy eating."

What is Mediterranean Diet?

When one reads the word Mediterranean, one tends to think nothing but of sea. Thinking of a vast sea brings to mind the sea food. When its history is looked into, it transpires that it has its roots in Mediterranean basin, a land which has been historically called a powerhouse of societal evolution of the world. As here the social history of whole world may be lying stored. This area in Nile valley was a good land for the people of East and West. The frequent interaction of people from different regions and culture had larger effect on customs, languages, religion, perspective, and had transformative effect on life style. This cultural integration and clash further had an effect on eating habit too.

Looking at the food content of Mediterranean diet one can see the reflection of diverse culture and class. Bread, wine and oil reflect village and agriculture; this is further complemented by vegetable like lettuce, mushroom, mallow and little preference for meat but much preference for fish and sea food. This shows the gluttonous nature of people from Rome. Here we also get Germanic flavour of pig's meat with garden vegetables. The beer was made with grains.

The food culture of bread, wine and oil went beyond Germanic and Christian Roman culture and entered the boundaries of Arabs. The reason was their existence at the southern shore of the Mediterranean. Their food culture was unique because of the variety of leafy vegetables they grew. They had egg plants, spinach, sugarcane, and fruits like oranges, citrus, lemon, and pomegranate and resembled rose water of the European cuisine. This had an influence on the cooking style of Latin and affect the recipes.

The big geographical event that is discovery of America by European has great additional impact on Mediterranean diet. This event added a range of new foodstuffs like beans, potatoes, tomatoes, chilli and peppers. Tomato, the red plant, was first ornamental and later was considered edible. It further became an important part of Mediterranean diet.

The historical analysis of Mediterranean diet shows how from feeding of Egyptian to discovery of America gave us the Mediterranean diet of the today. The nutritional model of Mediterranean diet is kept so much in high commendation that it is related to cultural, social, and environmental that it is intimately related to Mediterranean people, their lifestyle and history.

There are some established health and cultural platforms like UNESCO which define Mediterranean diet unfolding the meaning of word diet which has come from the word 'diata' that means lifestyle, a way of life. It focuses on the journey of food from landscape to the table; covering cuisine, harvesting, processing, preparation, fishing, cooking and a specific way of consumption.

There is a variation in Mediterranean diet in different countries due to ethnic and cultural differences, diverse religion and economic disparity. As per the description and recommendation of dietician and food experts the Mediterranean diet has the following proportion of foods. In cereals there are whole grains and legumes. For fats olive oil is a major source. Onion, garlic, tomatoes and leafy vegetables and peppers are major greens. Fresh fruits are major in snacks and desserts. Eggs, milk, yogurt and other dairy products are taken moderately. The food items like red meat, processed food, refined sugar are taken as little as possible.

This diet has 25 % to 35% proportion of fat content of the calorie count and saturated fat is never beyond 8 %. As far as oil is concerned there are region-wise alternatives. In central and northern Italy butter and lard are commonly used in cooking. Olive is mainly used for snacks and salad dressing.

This diet reflect food pattern of Crete, rest of Greece and much part of Italy in early 1960. It gained widespread recognition in 1990s. There is an irony in Mediterranean diet although people living in this region have a tendency to consume high amount of fats but they enjoy far better cardiovascular health as compared to people of America who consume equal amount of fat.

The tradition of Mediterranean diet offers cuisine rich in colour, taste, flavour and aroma. Most of all it keeps us closer to nature. It may be simple in looks but rich in health and has much to offer that is no way less than any other healthy diet. Some Americans describe Mediterranean diet as all styles of homemade pasta with Parmesan sauce and enrichment with a few pieces of meat is pretty occasional. That too for replacing beans and macaroni. It has omnipresence of so many fresh vegetables with just olive oil sprinkled. And desserts in this diet have nothing but always fresh fruits.

However, a good Mediterranean diet does not include ever soybean oil, canola or any other refined oil. There is no room for processed meat, refined sugar, white bread, refined grains or white pasta or pizza dough containing white flour.

This diet is characterised with a balanced use of food items which have high amount of fibre, unsaturated fats and antioxidants. Besides, there is an approach which gives health a priority by cutting the consumption of unhealthy animal fats and meat. This strikes a balance between the amount of energy intake and its consumption.

This magical diet is not just a preferential health food, with a wide range of magical recipes but also a conduit between wide ranges of cultures. People of this region are son of the soil and so is their food that comes from land and soil. It can ensure, if consumed rationally, efficacy of different bodily functions.

Some famous health organisations across the globe have designed food pyramids to make it clear what are the most common forms of Mediterranean region. It became popular among health activists because people of this region have high life expectancy despite less access to health facilities. It has been recommended by American Heart Association and American Diabetes Association that Mediterranean diet lowers the risk of cardiovascular disease and type two diabetes. If a patterned Mediterranean diet plan is followed, it may have a lasting effect on health and can help in reducing and maintaining healthy weight.

What are the benefits of Mediterranean Diet?

In this nutrition and health conscious world medical scientists, nutritionists and health scientists keep researching for healthy options and lifestyle changes which can ensure health and longevity along with agility. There is an emerging consensus among health experts that a diet which has fibre, balanced amount of protein, healthy fats and minerals can lead to optimum health and a healthy life.

It can check cardiovascular diseases, diabetes, cancer, stroke and help in maintaining healthy weight. Mediterranean diet has all these attributes. Its ingredients are rich in plants, healthy fats, fruits, whole grains, healthy meat and much more. As a matter of fact, it has all the elements which are essential to a healthy diet. There has been claims about its positive effect on health and physical well-being.

In a study conducted over 25000 women across a period of 12 years it has been established that those who consume Mediterranean diet has 25 percent less chances of having any cardiovascular

disease. The reason behind this positive change is decline in inflammation, glucose level in blood and an improved body mass index.

There is low saturated fat with high amount of monosaturated fats, protein and dietary fibre. Its olive oil has a major healthy element that is oleic acid. It is highly beneficial for the health of human heart. **It has the approval of European Food Safety Authority** Panel on Dietetic Products, Nutrition and Allergies. It has been mentioned that its polyphenols protects the oxidation of lipids in blood. It happens because of priority being given to olive oil which has oleic acid that helps in maintaining normal LDL level in blood and may check cardiovascular diseases. This has been claimed by American Heart Association as well that consumption of olive oil can be an aid to maintaining cardiovascular health. If this diet is followed the intake of refined breads, processed foods and unhealthy meat gets reduced, on the other hand it recommends replacing hard liquor with red wine. This way it can reduce the risk of cardiovascular diseases.

This diet has high fiber content. This reduces glucose level in blood and checks the causes which develop type 2 diabetes. This fiber makes one feel full and keep eating cravings under control.

This also helps in keeping weight under check and reduces constipation and helps regulate bowel movement.

Maintaining healthy weight is key factor to good health. It becomes easy to maintain an ideal weight when a fruit and vegetable rich diet is taken. The icing on the cake is total absence of refined sugar and white floor. A physical routine if is combined with it, it becomes easy to maintain a healthy weight. This may help in reducing obesity as well. Moreover, maintaining an ideal weight can give us multiple health benefits.

It has been found through a comprehensive research that a regular and monitored consumption of Mediterranean diet can reduce the risk of death from cancer by five to six percent. This has been confirmed in a study conducted on cancer patients in 2017. It has also been found that it may decrease the chances of cancer.

Stress is the key factor of affecting life adversely today. Mediterranean diet can be a relaxant here. It has been found in various studies that a sincere adherence to Mediterranean diet can check the impairment of cognitive ability. It does so by improving good cholesterol, levels of blood sugar and overall health of blood vessels. This as a result reduce your risk of dementia or Alzheimer's disease.

Mediterranean diet with maximum vegetables, fruits and nuts in it, is rich with antioxidants, vitamins and other nutrients. This helps cells form going through any damaging process. This damage otherwise occurs if there is an oxidative stress. Consequently, it reduces the risk of Parkinson's disease by fifty percent. Adhering to this diet can also lower the causes of depression and give a healthier state of mind.

It has been noticed in a study conducted by food scientists over women who had chances of stroke in United Kingdom. When they followed Mediterranean diet very strictly it reduced their chances of getting stroke by twenty percent. However, it was not so in men. But the clinical researches are underway to observe its effect on the male gender as well.

National Institute on Aging funded a small study on aging which was published on 2018. In the journal it was highlighted, how looking at brain scan of 70 persons it was found that the people who strictly adhered to Mediterranean diet did not show any sign of aging. While those who had preference for other forms of diet had a plaque pattern which adds the adverse effect of aging. This shows that Mediterranean diet adds longevity to human life and gives lasting health.

Lungs play an important role in oxygenating our body but with age its inhalation ability impairs. The whole grains, dairy products and fish can improve the ability of lungs to perform better. Further, those who remain disciplined and steadfast in taking Mediterranean diet has 22-29 percent less chances of getting hearing loss.

It is an obvious fact that Mediterranean diet has an ample amount of nutrients and if we consume this diet it helps in prevention of muscle damage and boost the muscle strength and enhances agility. This improves efficiency of brain. This means consumers of this diet have better thinking and learning abilities, an improved memory and much better concentration.

This diet is quite beneficial for kidney patients and those who for some reason have to undergo kidney transplant. In studies, it has been found that it can reduce the risk of kidney dysfunction. Further, it can bring down graft failure by as much as thirty two percent and its loss by twenty six percent in the patients who undergo kidney transplant.

If a person develops inflammatory bowel diseases like piles, Mediterranean diet can cause a cure. It has been found after studies and preparing case histories that consumer of this diet are 57 percent less prone to develop Crohn's disease.

How to get started?

The best way to cause a change is to start it. But the biggest question that always awaits its answer is the way to start. Nonetheless the situation is much better if what we are to start has multiple benefits. Mediterranean diet obviously falls in this category where advantages outnumber the limitations, it may force on our lifestyle.
If you feel that it is difficult to change your diet, you can choose alternatives which really work well and can help switching to healthier option. Here are certain ways that can help switch to Mediterranean diet.

It is good to start by keeping vegetables and fruits at the upper ladder in your list of priorities and giving sausages and pepperoni in salad dressing a backseat. You can start by giving a plate of tomato slices a try. It should be just given a drizzle of olive oil and meshed feta cheese. Soups, crudité plates and salads can be awesome starters.
Skipping breakfast may seem effective but it can put extra burden on your system to keep you going. On the contrary, whole grains, fruits and other foods which are rich in fibre can be an effective way to start your day. Moreover, it will keep you filled and your cravings at a bay.

Replacing usual calorie loaded desserts like cake, ice cream, pastries etc. with fruits like apples, grapes, fresh figs or strawberries. This will make you digest better and stay lighter. A refreshing feeling will work as a motivation and keep you adherent to this magical diet.
If you leap to change it may never happen. There is a famous saying, 'A thousand miles journey starts with a single step.' This is quite applicable to shifting to Mediterranean diet. You can start with small steps like sauté with olive oil, eat more vegetables and fruits by enjoying, in starter, some salad. Replace your snacks with fruits. Similarly, other heavy dishes can be substituted with veggies.

Preferring skimmed milk or milk with 2 percent fats over full fat milk. This will be making you feel lighter and healthier. As a result it will work as a motivating factor for opting Mediterranean diet. The change felt in energy level and the nutrition experienced will work as a triggering factor and a driving force.

It is said if it is easy, it is achievable. The most accessible is to use whole grains in place of refined grains. Your choice should be whole wheat bread and not white bread that is made of refined flour. Similarly, brown rice or wild rice should replace white rice. Sometimes it is difficult choose authentic whole grains. It is easy now as a black and gold stamp has been developed by Oldways Whole Grain Council to select quality over paste.

Ancient grains or whole grains form an important part of Mediterranean diet. There is a huge variety of these grains. These are amaranth, faro, millet, spelt, and the believably Egyptian, Kamut; yet another is teff, it is similar to poppy seed in its size. You can try one seed at a time. Slowly and steady you can move to more options. In other words, you can switch to the other variety of seeds. As each seed has its own flavour and texture. The good news is these whole grains have become quite popular and are quite common. Consequently, these are now available in mainstream restaurants as well. It means you can try it and then make it a part of your diet.

If you make up your mind to go for it. You should take at least six servings a day. Half of it should be of whole grains. It may be worrisome to some because of carbs. But you can throw your tension to winds because it, for sure, will cause long term benefits. You should not overlook the fact that quick loss of weight may not be healthy. So whole grain in Mediterranean diet is the best option.

You may not be able to swap your current diet with Mediterranean at once. So, one meal based on vegetables, whole grains and beans. Spices and herbs can be peppered with spices to add a palatable punch.

If you are protein conscious and remain worried about it in your diet. Your dependence on meat can end by giving room to lentils in your diet. As these are the sources of high protein and have much fibre too. Beans have an edge, as these have ample antioxidants too. How motivating!

If it is in your easy reach, it can be your easy preference. Stocking your pantry with handy ingredients. These ingredients should be easy to use. Some of these can be popular protein sources like lentils, chickpeas and beans. Lentils have only twenty five minutes of cooking time without any need of overnight soaking. As for chickpeas and canned beans, you only need to rinse and then you can just put them into soups, burgers, salads, sandwiches and much more.

Giving up meat altogether may be a challenge but you can give it a start by taking meat in small proportion. Using small pieces of chicken or lean meat slices. You can stir fry your dish and avoid deep fry. It will keep it less oil soaked and more nourishing. It is a good news for fish eater as when they are on Mediterranean diet they can eat two servings of salmon, sardines and tuna these are essential to Mediterranean diet at least twice a week. There may be a risk of mercury but in the opinion of American nutritionists here benefits outrun the risk. The variety of fish mentioned here has comparatively less amount of mercury.

Dairy products are also a great protein source. Yogurt if it is Greek and a cheese cube is something which those on Mediterranean diet are encouraged to eat. But it should be in moderation.

In short, Mediterranean diet is a healthy option with wide range of tasty choices. If you start with an easy approach taking small steps at a time. Making little changes in your meal plans, you can go a long way.

21 Days Meal Plan

DAYS	Breakfast	Lunch	Snacks	Dinner
Day 1	Spinach and Artichoke Frittata	Mediterranean Chickpea Quinoa Bowl	15 Minute Mediterranean Chickpea Salad	Mediterranean Portobello Mushroom Pizzas with Arugula Salad
Day 2	Hearty Breakfast Fruit Salad	Harissa Chickpea Stew With Eggplant and Millet	Lemon Herb Mediterranean Pasta Salad	Slow-Cooker Mediterranean Quinoa with Arugula
Day 3	Shakshuka	Five-Minute Heirloom Tomato Toast	Hummus	Walnut-Rosemary Crusted Salmon
Day 4	Balsamic Berries with Honey Yogurt	Eggplant and Herb Flatbread	Mini Greek Pita Pizzas	Mediterranean Stuffed Chicken Breasts
Day 5	Caprese Avocado Toast	15-Minute Mediterranean Couscous with Tuna and Pepperoncini	Healthy Avocado Cilantro White Bean Dip	Charred Shrimp & Pesto Buddha Bowls
Day 6	Spinach Feta Breakfast Wraps	Pesto Quinoa Bowls With Roasted Veggies and Labneh	Homemade Granola Bars Recipe (Gluten-Free, Vegan, Dairy-Free)	Sheet-Pan Salmon with Sweet Potatoes & Broccoli

Day 7	Easy Homemade Muesli	Greek Yogurt Chicken Salad Stuffed Peppers	Peach Caprese Skewers	Greek Cauliflower Rice Bowls with Grilled Chicken
Day 8	Kale and Goat Cheese Frittata Cups	15-Minute Mezze Plate with Toasted Za'atar Pita Bread	Charcuterie Bistro Lunch Box	Prosciutto Pizza with Corn & Arugula
Day 9	Easy, Fluffy Lemon Ricotta Pancakes	Greek Lemon Chicken Skewers With Tzatziki Sauce	Hummus, Feta & Bell Pepper Cracker	Vegan Mediterranean Lentil Soup
Day 10	Smashed Egg Toasts with Herby Lemon Yogurt	Eggplant Pizza	Tomato-Basil Skewers	BBQ Shrimp with Garlicky Kale & Parmesan - Herb Couscous
Day 11	Mediterranean Breakfast Pitas	Cold Lemon Zooldes	Marinated Olives & Feta	Green Shakshuka with Spinach, Chard & Feta
Day 12	Crispy White Beans with Greens and Poached Egg	Stuffed Eggplant	Garlic Hummus	One-Skillet Salmon with Fennel & Sun-Dried Tomato Couscous
Day 13	Breakfast Grain Salad with Blueberries, Hazelnuts & Lemon	Wild Alaska Salmon and Smashed Cucumber Grain Bowls	Clementine & Pistachio Ricotta	Chicken & Spinach Skillet Pasta with Lemon & Parmesan
Day 14	Eggs with Summer Tomatoes, Zucchini, and Bell Peppers	Harissa Potato Salad	Ricotta & Yogurt Parfait	Baked chicken and Ricotta Meatballs
Day 15	Avocado and Egg Breakfast Pizza	Greek Lemon Chicken Soup	Mediterranean Picnic Snacks	Chickpea Vegetable Coconut Curry
Day 16	Mediterranean Breakfast Sandwich	Mediterranean Bento Lunch	Crock Pot Chunky Monkey Paleo Trail Mix Recipe	Broccoli Rabe and Burrata with Lemon
Day 17	Breakfast Hash with Brussels sprouts and Sweet Potatoes	Greek Meatball Mezze Bowls	Savory Feta Spinach and Sweet Red Pepper Muffins	Tomato Poached Cod with Special Herbs
Day 18	Mediterranean Keto Low Carb Egg Muffins with Ham	Mediterranean Chicken with Orzo Salad	Smoked Salmon, Avocado and Cucumber Bites	Chickpea Shawarma Salad
Day 19	Spinach and Artichoke Frittata	Mediterranean Chickpea Quinoa Bowl	15 Minute Mediterranean Chickpea Salad	Mediterranean Portobello Mushroom Pizzas with Arugula Salad
Day 20	Hearty Breakfast Fruit Salad	Harissa Chickpea Stew With Eggplant and Millet	Lemon Herb Mediterranean Pasta Salad	Slow-Cooker Mediterranean Quinoa with Arugula
Day 21	Shakshuka	Five-Minute Heirloom Tomato Toast	Hummus	Walnut-Rosemary Crusted Salmon

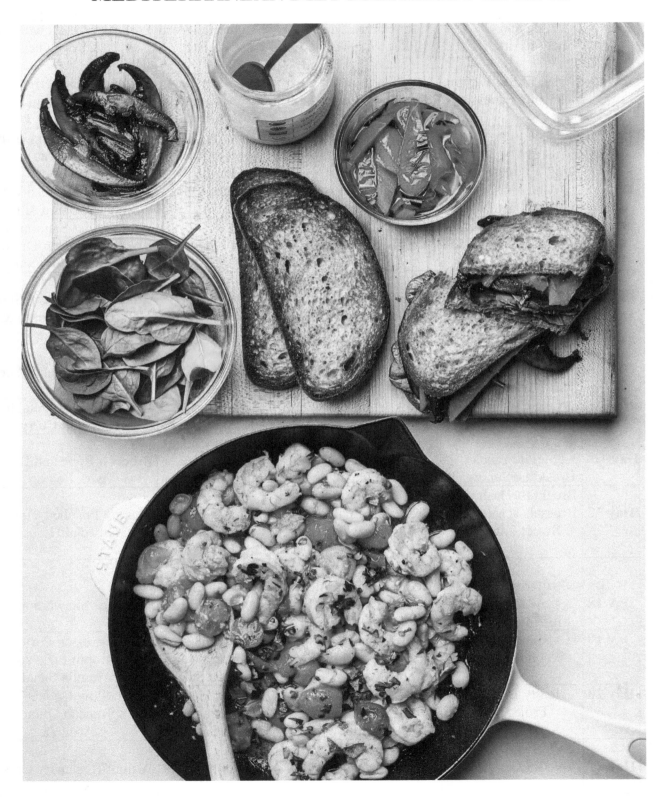

Spinach and Artichoke Frittata

Serving size: 4
Servings per recipe: 2
Calories: 316
Preparation time: 5 minutes
Cooking time: 22 – 25 minutes

Ingredients:

- large eggs 10
- full-fat sour cream ½
- Dijon mustard 1 tbs
- kosher salt 1 tsp
- freshly ground black pepper 1/4 teaspoon
- grated Parmesan cheese (about 3 ounces), divided 1
- cup olive oil 2 tablespoons
- marinated artichoke hearts, drained, patted dry, and quartered About 14 ounces
- baby spinach 5 ounces
- 2 cloves garlic, minced

Nutrition Information: based on 6 servings
Carb: 6.4 g
Protein: 17.9 g
Fats: 25.9 g

Instructions:

1. Place a rack in centre of the oven set temperature at 400˚c.
2. In a large bowl put sour cream, mustard, pepper salt and half cup of Parmesan cheese, stir with a whisk well until well combined; keep at a side.
3. Take a skillet of about 10" skillet (non-stick or cast iron) heat oil over mediuk flame. Put artichoke in a layer, cook stir in between, till light brown, not more than 8 minutes. Now spinach and garlic is to be added, toss it is wilted till liquid evaporates.
4. After spreading the mixture evenly in a layer, pour the mixture of egg over vegetables. Sprinkle 1/2 cup of Parmesan. For setting the eggs well over veggies tilt it. Cook for 2-3 minutes or till the time the eggs settle.
5. Bake for 13-15 minutes. Cut in the centre of frittata to check even cooking. Leave it for five minutes to cool, slice into wedges shape.

Hearty Breakfast Fruit Salad

Serving size: 1
Servings per recipe: 5
Calories: 282
Preparation time: 10 minutes
Cooking time: 1 hour 20 minutes

Ingredients:

- pearl or hulled barley or any sturdy whole grain 1 cup
- water 3 cups
- olive oil, divided 3 tablespoons
- kosher salt 1/2 teaspoon
- 1/2 large pineapple, peeled and cut into 1 1/2- to 2-inch chunks (2 to 2 1/2 cups)
- medium tangerines or mandarin 6 , or large oranges 5(about 1 1/2 pounds total)
- pomegranate seeds 1 1/4 cups
- small bunch fresh mint 1

For the dressing:

- honey or another sweetener 1/3 cup
- Juice and finely grated zest of 1 lemon (about 1/4 cup juice)
- Juice and finely grated zest of 2 limes (about 1/4 cup juice)
- kosher salt 1/2 teaspoon
- olive oil 1/4 cup
- toased hazelnut or nut oil 1/4 cup

Nutrition Information

Carbs: 34.8 g

Proteins: 3.7 g

Fats: 16.6 g

Instructions

1. With a parchment paper line rimmed baking sheets. In a strainer wash barley under cold water till the water below is clear for around one minute. Shake the strainer gently to drain off the excess water. On one of the prepared baking sheets place barley and using spatula spread out the grains into a single layer. Leave it be completely dry for 3-4 minutes.
2. In a microwave or stove top warm the water, keep it aside.
3. In a medium saucepan heat 2 tablespoon oil on high heat till simmering. Add barely carefully and toast, keep stirring constantly, till they darken a bit. It generally takes 1 minute to 90 seconds.

4. Add salt and warm water and bring it to boil. Turn the heat to simmer to the lowest, cover the pan and keep cooking until soft and most of the water has been absorbed, for around 40-50 minutes. Take the pot off the heat and leave it covered for 10 minutes, this way the barley would steam and finish absorbing water. By that time prepare mint, fruit and dressing.

5. Into one of the large containers place the pineapple chunks. Peel and cut mandarins, tangerines, or oranges into segments, remove as much of the bitter white pith as possible. Place these fruits in another container, cover and refrigerate. Keep pomegranate seeds in a covered box separately and refrigerate.

6. Mince or slice the mint leaves thinly. Keep it in a covered container and refrigerator.

7. In a medium bowl whisk juice, honey, zest and salt together. Mizzle in olive oil, nut oil, while whisking constantly until incorporated. You can cover and refrigerate or refrigerate in a jar.

8. Shift the cooked barley onto the second prepared baking sheet and spread in a layer evenly. Leave to cool completely. For around 10-20 minutes. Mizzle barley with leftover 1 tablespoon of oil and mix to coat.

9. Shift barley to a large container. Cover the container and keep in a refrigerator.

10. At the time of serving, scoop 2/3 cup of barley into each bowl. In each bowl add six pieces of pineapple, 10-12 orange segments, and with it ¼ cup pomegranate seeds into each bowl. Now add 1-2 tablespoons of the mint and 2-3 tablespoons of dressing to each bowl. Stir in order to mix and coat it with the dressing.

Shakshuka

Serving size: 4
Servings per recipe: 6
Calories: 146
Preparation time: 10
Cooking time: 25 to 30 minutes

Ingredients:

- *whole peeled tomatoes 1 (28-ounce) can*
- *olive oil 2 tablespoons*
- *finely chopped small yellow onion 1*
- *tomato paste 2 tablespoons*
- *Harissa 1 tablespoon*
- *garlic, minced 3 cloves*
- *ground cumin 1 teaspoon*
- *kosher salt 1/2 teaspoon*
- *large eggs 6*
- *loosely packed chopped fresh cilantro leaves and tender stems 1/4 cup feta cheese, crumbled (about 1/2 cup, optional 2 ounces*

Nutrition Information based on 10 servings
Carb: 7.8 g
Protein: 7.9 g
Fats: 9.7 g

Instructions

1. In a large bowl pour tomatoes as well as their juice. Crush with hands carefully, pieces should be bite-sized.
2. In a skillet heat oil for 10-12 minutes on medium flame. Now add onion sauté for 5 minutes or till soft. Put harissa, garlic, cumin, tomato paste and salt. Sauté until aromatic.
3. After adding tomatoes simmer till sauce gets slightly thickens. (10 minutes)
4. Now remove skillet from stove. Make small six holes in sauce and crack an egg into each.
5. Spoon a little sauce over each egg. If you expose the yolks, white of egg cooks faster.
6. For even cooking of eggs keep rotating the pan or till the time white sets. It generally takes 8 to 12 minutes.
7. Remove the pan from flame. Sprinkle feta and cilantro. Your dish is ready to be served with bread or fita.

Caprese Avocado Toast

Serving size: 2
Servings per recipe: 2
Calories: 649
Preparation time: 4 minutes
Cooking time: 7-8 minutes

Ingredients:

- slices hearty sandwich bread, such as peasant bread, sourdough, whole-wheat or multi-grain- 2
- medium avocado, halved and pit removed- 1
- grape tomatoes, halved- 8
- fresh *ciliegine* or bite-sized mozzarella balls 2 ounces (about 12)
- large fresh basil leaves, torn 4

  balsamic glaze 2 tablespoons

Nutrition Information
Carb: 86.4 g
Protein: 23.9 g
Fats: 24.6 g

Instructions

1. First toaste the bread. Meanwhile mash avocado in a small-sized bowl.
2. Over the toast mashed spread avocado. Use tomatoes, mozzarella balls and basil leaves for topping each slice. Thereafter sprinkle balsamic glaze. Serve at once.

Spinach Feta Breakfast Wraps

Serving size: 4
Servings per recipe: 4
Calories: 543
Preparation time: 10 minutes
Cooking time: 12 minutes

Ingredients:

- large eggs 10
- baby spinach 1/2 pound
- whole-wheat tortillas 4
- cherry or grape tomatoes, halved 1/2 pint
- feta cheese, crumbled 4 ounces
- Butter or olive oil   1 teaspoon
- Salt   ¼ tsp.
- Pepper   ¼ tsp.

Nutrition Information 4 servings
Carbs: 46.5 g
Protein: 28.1 g
Fats: 27 g

Instructions:

1. Stir the eggs well to combine the white and yolks. Coat skillet's bottom with teaspoon of olive oil and place on medium flame. At the melting of butter or heating of oil drain the eggs in skillet, stir in between till the eggs are cooked. Add a pinch of salt with black pepper. Slide the material to a platter, cool at room temperature.
2. Rinse the skillet, now put it on medium flame, and add another teaspoon of oil or butter. Add spinach. Keep stirring until the spinach is limp. Spread wilted spinach on a plate, cool it at room temperature.
3. On a surface arrange a tortilla. Add spinach, tomatoes, feta and quarter of the eggs in mid of tortilla, wrap tightly. Repeat the same procedure with the rest of the tortillas. In a gallon zip-top bag place the wraps and freeze till ready to eat.
4. If you want to freeze longer than a week. In an aluminium foil wrap burritos, it will prevent the freezer from burning. Reheat in microwave on high for 2 minutes.

Easy Homemade Muesli

Serving size: 1
Servings per recipe: 8
Calories: 275
Preparation time: 15 minutes
Cooking time: 15 minutes

Ingredients:

- rolled oats- 3 1/2 cups
- wheat bran- 1/2 cup
- kosher salt- 1/2 teaspoon
- ground cinnamon- 1/2 teaspoon
- sliced almonds- 1/2 cup
- raw pecans, coarsely chopped- 1/4 cup
- raw pepitas (shelled pumpkin seeds)- 1/4 cup
- unsweetened coconut flakes-1/2 cup
- dried apricots, coarsely chopped-1/4 cup
- dried cherries-1/4 cup

Nutrition Information: Carbs: 36 g; Protein: 8.5 g; Fats: 13.4 g

Instructions

1. To divide the oven into thirds, arrange two racks and heat to 350 °F. Put wheat bran, salt, cinnamon and oats on a rimmed baking sheet. Spread an even layer. On the second rimmed baking sheet put pecans, pepitas, and almonds, to combine toss, spread evenly in a layer. Both baking sheets should be transferred to oven, keeping oats on top part of the rack and at bottom nuts.
2. Set aside the baking sheet having nuts in order to cool. Spatter coconut powder over oats. Bake the upper rack till coconut is golden brown, preferably 5 minutes. Remove from, cool for 10 minutes.
3. Shift the material of both the baking sheets into a large bowl.
4. Put cherries and apricots, to combine well; toss.
5. You can store muesli in airtight container at room temperature for a month.
6. You can have it with cereals, yogurt, and oatmeal or with drops of honey.

Kale and Goat Cheese Frittata Cups

Serving size: 1 cup
Servings per recipe: 8 cups
Calories: 179
Preparation time: 5 minutes
Cooking time: 35-40 minutes

Ingredients:

- chopped lacinato kale 2 cups
- garlic clove, thinly sliced 1
- olive oil 3 tablespoons
- red pepper flakes 1/4 teaspoon
- large eggs 8
- Salt 1/4 teaspoon
- ground black pepper Dash
- dried thyme 1/2 teaspoon
- goat cheese, crumbled 1/4 cup

Nutrition Information

Carbs: 1.2 g

Protein: 10.0 g

Fats: 14.7 g

Instructions

1. Oven is to be preheated to 350°F. Remove the leaves from kale ribs for getting to cups of kale. Now wash and leave the leaves to dry. Next cut these leaves into half inch wide strips.
2. Cook garlic in a non-tick skillet, preferably of 10 inch, in one tablespoon of oil. Keep the flame at medium to high level for 30 seconds. Now add kale and red pepper flakes, keep cook until soft. Generally it takes around 2 minutes.
3. Beat eggs along with salt and pepper in a medium sized bowl. Now thyme and kale are to be added to the blended mixture.
4. Grease a 12 cup muffin tin with 2 tablespoon olive oil. The tops are to be spattered with goat cheese. Bake for 25-30 minutes or these are set in the centre.
5. It tastes best if eaten warm. You can refrigerate the leftovers. But consume within a week.

Easy, Fluffy Lemon Ricotta Pancakes

Serving size: 4
Servings per recipe: 12
Calories: 344
Preparation time: 10 minutes
Cooking time: 15-18 minutes

Ingredients:

- large eggs 4
- medium lemon 1
- whole-milk ricotta cheese 1 cup
- whole or 2% milk 1/2 cup
- all-purpose flour 1 cup
- granulated sugar 1 tablespoon
- baking powder 1 teaspoon
- kosher salt 1/4 teaspoon
- Unsalted butter, for cooking 1 tablespoon

Nutrition Information
Carbs: 32.3 g
Protein: 17.7 g
Fats: 15.9 g

Instructions

1. Mix white and yolk of the 4 large eggs with an electric hand mixer in a medium sized bowl.
2. Grate zest and a medium sized lemon over the yolks, squeeze lemon juice into the bowl. Now add 1/2 whole or 2 % milk, 1 cup whole-milk ricotta cheese, whisk to combine. Next add 1 cup all-purpose flour, 1 teaspoon baking powder, sugar (granulated) ¼ teaspoon kosher salt, and mix well to combine.
3. On mid-high speed beat egg whites until stiff peaks form. 1/3 of beaten egg whites stirred into yolk batter using rubber spatula. Gently fold the left egg whites to combine well.
4. On medium flame heat a non-stick skillet. Coat with 1 teaspoon unsalted butter. Put batter into pan ¼ of cup, at a time 3. You can use spatula to spread a round of 4" each. Keep cooking till the surface bubbles appear, edges look dry and bottom turns golden brown, flip and cook till it is golden brown.
5. Pancakes can now be transferred to a warm plate or oven.

Smashed Egg Toasts with Herby Lemon Yogurt

Serving size: 4
Servings per recipe: 4
Calories: 437
Preparation time: 5 minutes
Cooking time: 15 minutes

Ingredients:

- large eggs 8
- garlic 1 clove
- medium lemon 1
- finely chopped fresh basil leaves, plus more for garnish 2 tablespoons
- finely chopped fresh dill, plus more for garnish 2 tablespoons finely
- chopped fresh chives, plus more for garnish 2 tablespoons plain
- Greek yogurt 2 cups

  extra-virgin olive oil, plus more for drizzling 2
- tablespoons kosher salt, plus more for sprinkling 3/4
- teaspoon
- freshly ground black pepper, plus more for sprinkling 1/2
- teaspoon country or sourdough bread (about 1-inch thick) 4 large
- slices unsalted butter, divided 4 tablespoons

Nutrition Information: Carbs: 7.4 g; **Protein:** 23.5 g; **Fats:** 35.5 g

Instructions

1. Fill quarter of a large pan with water, boil on high flame, fill another large bowl with ice and cold water. Lower heat to simmer. Lower 8 eggs gently, one at a time. Boil for 6.30 minutes. Now transfer eggs to ice bath, after 2 minutes, peel eggs under running water.
2. Grate the zest 1 medium sized lemon finely, squeeze and extract juice, mince garlic clove. Chop basil leaf to have 2 tablespoon leaves and same amount of fresh dill and fresh chives. Add 2 cups yogurt (Greek) and 2 tablespoon extra-virgin olive oil, ¾ teaspoon kosher salt and ½ teaspoon black pepper. Whisk to combine.
3. Cut 4 slices (1") of a crusty bread. Melt 2 tablespoon unsalted butter in skillet of large size on medium flame. Add 2 slices, cook till crisp and golden brown. Shift to a large platter.
4. On bread slices spread yogurt mixture, top with 2 eggs. With back of a spoon, gently smash eggs. Spatter black pepper, kosher salt and herbs, you can sprinkle a little more olive oil.

Mediterranean Breakfast Pitas

Serving size: 1 filled pita
Servings per recipe: 4
Calories: 206
Preparation time: 5 minutes
Cooking time: 15 -20 minutes

Ingredients:

- large eggs, at room temperature- 4
- Salt to taste
- whole-wheat pita breads with pockets, cut in half 1/2 cup
- hummus 1 (4 ounces)
- medium cucumber, thinly sliced into rounds 2
- large dice medium tomatoes,
- fresh parsley leaves, coarsely chopped Handful
- Freshly ground black pepper
- Hot sauce (optional)

Nutrition Information
Carbs: 22.9 g
Proteins: 12 g
Fats: 8.3 g

Instructions

1. Pour water in medium sized pan to the full. Bring water to boil. Place room temperature eggs in this water and cook for around 7 minutes. Next drain the hot water and place the eggs under running tap of cold water. Now peel these eggs and make slices of ¼ inch thickness. Sprinkle salt.
2. Now spread 2 tablespoons of hummus inside each pita. Now put diced tomatoes and cucumber slices into every pita. Salt and pepper are to be sprinkled now. In each pita tuck a sliced egg and sprinkle with hot sauce and parsley.

Crispy White Beans with Greens and Poached Egg

Serving size: 4
Servings per recipe: 2
Calories: 301
Preparation time: 5 minutes
Cooking time: 15 minutes

Ingredients:

- olive oil, divided 3 tablespoons
- can cannellini beans, drained and rinsed 1 (15-ounce)
- kosher salt, divided 1 teaspoon
- za'atar, divided 2 teaspoons
- medium bunch Swiss chard (about 10 ounces), stems removed and leaves thinly sliced- 1
- garlic, minced 2 cloves
- red pepper flakes, plus more for serving 1/4
- teaspoon freshly squeezed lemon juice 1 tablespoon
- large eggs, poached 4

Nutrition Information
Carbs: 26.5 g
Proteins: 15.5 g
Fats: 15.5 g

Instructions

1. In a large frying pan heat 2 tablespoon oil over medium heat. Keep until shimmering. Spread the beans into an even layer, cook until light brown at bottom. it generally takes 2-4 minutes. Add 1 teaspoon za'tar and ½ teaspoon salt. Stir to combine. Beans are to be spread again and cooked, keep stirring till beans turn golden brown and bubbled on all sides.
2. Put rest of 1 tablespoon oil on the pan. Add chard, rest of half teaspoon salt and 1 teaspoon za'atar, red pepper flakes and garlic. Stir in between and keep cooking until the chard gets soft. Take the pan off the flame, put lemon juice, to combine well toss.
3. In 4 bowls divide beans and greens, top each with a poached egg and a bit more of red pepper flakes.

Breakfast Grain Salad with Blueberries, Hazelnuts & Lemon

Serving size: 2
Servings per recipe: 8
Calories: 353
Preparation time: 5 minutes
Cooking time: 25 minutes

Ingredients:

- steel-cut oats 1 cup
- dry golden quinoa 1 cup
- dry millet 1/2 cup
- olive oil, divided 3 tablespoons
- piece fresh ginger, peeled and cut into coins- 1 (1-inch)
- large lemons, zest and juice 2
- maple syrup 1/2 cup
- Greek yogurt (or soy yogurt, if you want to make this vegan) 1 cup
- Nutmeg 1/4 teaspoon
- hazelnuts, roughly chopped and toasted 2 cups
- blueberries or mixed berries   2 cups

Nutrition Information

Carbs: 38 g

Proteins: 9.3 g

Fats: 20.1 g

Instructions

1. In a fine mesh strainer mix millet, oats and quinoa. For a minute rinse under running water. Keep aside.
2. Over medium flame in a 3 quart saucepan heat one tablespoon olive oil. Put rinsed millet, oats and quinoa. Cook for 2-3 minutes. Add 4 ½ cups of water and stir ¾ salt, zest of a lemon and ginger coins.
3. Bring the water to boil, after covering turn the heat down and simmer for about 20 minutes. Turn the burner off and leave for 5 minutes, remove the lid and touch lightly with a fork. Take the ginger off. On a large baking sheet spread grains allow it cool for minimum half an hour.
4. With a spoon put the cooled grain into a large bowl. The zest of second lemon is stirred in.
5. Whisk the remaining olive oil (2 tablespoons) in a mid-sized bowl with juice of 2 lemons, wait till emulsified. Mix yogurt, maple syrup and nutmeg. Flow this into grains and stir unit coated well. Add in blueberries and hazelnuts. Try taste and flavour with salt, if required. For better flavour refrigerate overnight.

Eggs with Summer Tomatoes, Zucchini, and Bell Peppers

Serving size: 1
Servings per recipe: 2
Calories: 226
Preparation time: 5 minutes
Cooking time: 30-35 minutes

Ingredients:

- olive oil 1 tablespoon
- small yellow onion, halved and thinly sliced 1
- garlic, minced 1 clove
- medium summer squash or zucchini (approximately 4 cups) 2
- medium tomatoes, chopped (approximately 3 cups) 2
- fresh thyme (optional) 1/2 teaspoon
- ground Spanish piquillo pepper or Spanish paprika 1 teaspoon
- medium red bell pepper 1
- Salt and pepper 1 tablespoon each
- large eggs 2

Nutrition Information based on 2 serving

Carbs: 20.6 g

Proteins: 11.1 g

Fats: 12.5 g

Instructions

1. In a large heavy skillet heat olive oil at medium heat. Add sliced onions, keep stirring to the point translucence. Next put garlic and cook for a minute. Next add squash and cook for 10 minutes or till soft. Then add, thyme (optional) and piquillo and allow to simmer to the point of even cooking and it turns stewy, for around 20 minutes.
2. Keep cooking ratatouille, meanwhile on the stovetop roast the pepper. Once cool, take off the core and seed, cut into 1'' pieces. Now put the skillet off the flame, add roasted peppers and put pepper and salt as per your taste. It is best to serve the dish warm.
3. You fry or boil eggs as per your choice. Divide veggie in two plates and add topping of eggs. You can serve it with buttered toast.

Avocado and Egg Breakfast Pizza

Serving size: 1
Servings per recipe: 4
Calories: 337
Preparation time: 10 minutes
Cooking time: 15 minutes

Ingredients:

- large Hass avocado 1
- finely chopped cilantro 1 tablespoon
- lime juice 1 ½ teaspoons
- salt 1/8 teaspoon
- pizza dough, homemade 1/2 pound
- Large eggs 4
- vegetable oil 1 tablespoon
- Hot sauce, for serving (optional)

Nutrition Information

Carbs: 33.2 g

Proteins: 12.3 g

Fats: 17.6 g

Instructions

1. Half lengthwise cut avocado, after removing pit, with a spoon scoop the flesh and put into a bowl. Now add lemon juice, cilantro and salt. With a few pieces of avocado, mash using a fork until smooth. Taste and adjust the flavour. If avocado is bigger more salt and lime juice may be required.
2. Divide dough in 4 pieces of equal size. Now roll each piece into a slim 6" circle. Try again if dough does not stay at a point.
3. Over a medium flame heat a well-seasoned cast iron skillet. Now place in the centre of the skillet one dough circle. For 1-2 minutes cook or till the underside is brown and the upper side is bubbly. Repeat procedure by flipping the dough circle. Press with spatula if puffing is seen in dough top. It may seem burnt in spots but it's ok. Transfer to platter and repeat with the left dough circles.
4. On each cooked piece of dough spread the avocado mixture.
5. Over the medium flame heat oil in the skillet. Now fry eggs to desired level and place it on top of pizza. Serve at once with hot sauce or without it.

Mediterranean Breakfast Sandwich

Serving size: 1
Servings per recipe: 4
Calories: 242
Preparation time: 15 minutes
Cooking time: 5 minutes

Ingredients:

- Multigrain sandwich thins 4
- Olive oil 4 teaspoons
- Snipped fresh rosemary 1 tablespoon or dried rosemary ½ teaspoon
- Eggs 4
- Fresh baby spinach leaves 2 cups
- Medium tomato cut into 8 slices- 1
- Reduced-fat feta cheese 4 tablespoons
- Kosher salt 1/8 teaspoon
- Freshly ground black pepper

Nutrition Information

Carbs: 25 g

Proteins: 13 g

Fats: 11.7 g

Instructions

1. Heat the oven beforehand to 375 degrees F. Now split sandwich thin, next brush cut sides using 2 teaspoons of the olive oil. keep the toast on baking sheet and put in oven for about 5 minutes or till the edges are light brown and crispy.
2. Over medium-high heat 2 teaspoons olive oil and over medium heat the rosemary. Break eggs, one at a time, into skillet. Cook until white are set but yolks are quite runny or for 1 minute. With spatula break yolks. Change side of eggs cook on other side till done. Take off from heat.
3. Now place the bottom half of the toasted sandwich on the 4 serving plates. Divide spinach among sandwich thins on plates. Do toppings of each with tomato slices, an egg, and 1 tablespoon of feta cheese. Sprinkle with pepper and salt. Now top it with the other sandwich thin halves.

Breakfast Hash with Brussels Sprouts and Sweet Potatoes

Serving Size:1
Servings per recipe: 4
Calories: 206
Preparation Time: 10 minutes
Cooking time: 25

Ingredients:

SWEET POTATO & BRUSSELS

- medium-large sweet potato, chopped into bite-size pieces (skin on) -1
- Brussels sprouts (quartered if large, halved if small) 3 cups
- avocado oil (or other neutral oil // or sub water if avoiding oil) 1 Tbsp.
- each sea salt and black pepper- 1 healthy pinch

THE REST

- avocado oil (or other neutral oil // or sub water if avoiding oil) 2 tsp.
- medium yellow, white, or red onion, finely chopped 1/2
- minced garlic cloves , 3
- finely diced Fuji or Jonagold apple (peeling optional // seeds + stem removed) 3/4 cup
- fresh minced sage (or sub dried) 1 Tbsp.
- dried currants (*optional*) 2 Tbsp.
  spicy chicken or pork sausage (*optional* // buy local and organic meat- 1 cup
- whenever possible // or sub Vegan Sausage) fresh spinach-2 heaping cups
- large eggs (farm fresh or organic, free range / pasture raised whenever possible // see notes for vegan options*) -4

Nutrition Information: Carbs: 19.3 g; Protein: 9.7 g; Fats: 11 g

Instruction

1. With a parchment paper line a baking sheet and preheat oven to 400 degrees F.

2. Put Brussels and sweet potato on baking sheet. Mizzle oil, flavour with pepper and salt and toss for coating. Bake for 22-28 minutes. Toss at mid-point for even cooking.

3. By that time over medium flame heat a large skillet. Once it is hot put oil and onion. Sauté for around a minute. Thereafter add apple, garlic, sage and currants. Sauté for around 3 minutes or to the point of turning golden brown and aromatic—stir in-between.

4. Add sausage and keep sautéing till golden brown and thoroughly cooked—5-8 minutes. Stir constantly and use spoon to break sausage in small pieces.

5. If sausage is cooked, put spinach, cover skillet and cook for a few minutes until tender. Add in and stir roasted Brussel sprouts and sweet potato. Turn off heat and keep aside until serving.

6. By that time over a medium flame heat a separate skillet. After it is hot add the number of eggs as per desire.

7. In the pan crack egg and cook for 3 minutes uncovered, after covering with a lid leave for 1-2 minutes to help the white cook and keep the yolk soft.

8. Garnish with hot sauce and fresh herbs. Store cooled down leftover kept covered in the fridge for 3-4 days. In freezer in can be kept for a month.

Mediterranean Keto Low Carb Egg Muffins with Ham

Serving size: 2
Servings per recipe: 6
Calories: 109 kcal
Preparation time: 10
Cooking time: 15

Ingredients:

- Slices of thin cut deli ham 9
- Canned roasted red pepper, sliced + additional for garnish 1/2 Cup
- Fresh spinach, minced 1/3 Cup
- Feta cheese, crumbled 1/4 Cup
- Large eggs 5
- Pinch of salt
- Pinch of pepper
- Pesto sauce 1 1/2 Tbsp.
- Fresh basil for garnish

Nutrition information

Carbs: 1.8 g

Protein: 9.3 g

Fats: 6.7 g

Instructions

1. Fore-heat oven to 400 F. profusely spray a muffin tin with cooking spray.
2. With each piece of muffin tin is to be lined with 1.5 pieces of ham, ensure that no place is left for egg mixture to fall out.
3. In the bottom of each muffin tin put a little bit of red pepper.
4. On the top of each red pepper put 1 tablespoon of minced spinach.
5. Do topping of pepper and spinach off with a heaping ½ tablespoon of crumbled feta cheese.
6. Whisk the eggs, salt and pepper. Now divide mixture of eggs equally among 6 muffin tins.
7. Bake till the eggs are puffy and are set for around 15-17 minutes.
8. After removing each cup from the tin of muffin, garnish it with ¼ teaspoon of pesto sauce, additionally, you can ass roasted red pepper slices and fresh basil.

Mediterranean Diet Lunch Recipes

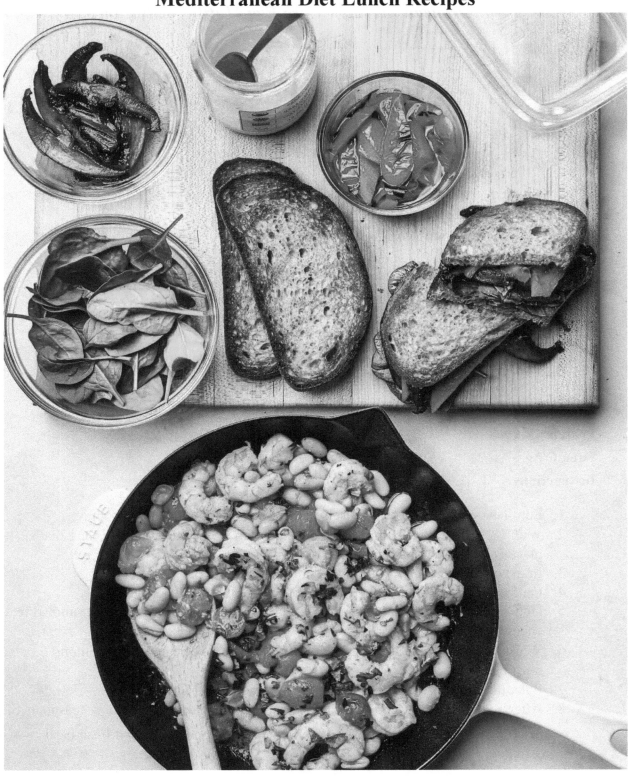

Mediterranean Chickpea Quinoa Bowl

Serving size: 1
Servings per recipe: 4
Calories: 479
Preparation time: 5 minutes
Cooking time: 20 minutes

Ingredients:

- jar roasted red peppers, rinsed- 1 (7 ounce)
- slivered almonds ¼ cup
- extra-virgin olive oil, divided 4 tablespoons
- garlic, minced 1 small clove
- paprika 1 teaspoon
- ground cumin ½ teaspoon
- crushed red pepper ¼ teaspoon (optional)
- cooked quinoa 2 cups
- Kalamata olives, chopped ¼ cup
- finely chopped red onion ¼ cup
- chickpeas, rinsed 15 ounce
- diced cucumber 1 cup
- crumbled feta cheese ¼ cup
- finely chopped fresh parsley 2 tablespoons

Nutrition Information 1 ½ cup
Carbs: 49.5 g

Proteins: 12.7 g

Fats: 24.8 g

Instructions

1. In a mini food processor place garlic, paprika, almonds, 2 tablespoon oil, cumin, crushed red pepper. Keep blending until much smooth.
2. In a medium bowl combine olives, red onion, quinoa and left 2 tablespoon oil.
3. At the time of serving divide quinoa mix into 4 bowls and top each with same amount of cucumber, chickpeas and red pepper sauce. Add parsley and feta.

Tomato Salad with Grilled Halloumi and Herbs

Serving size: 1
Servings per recipe: 4 servings
Calories: 197
Preparation time: 8 minutes
Cooking time: 2 minutes

Ingredients:

- tomatoes, sliced into rounds 1 pound
- lemon ½
- Flaky salt and freshly ground pepper
- Extra-virgin olive oil
- halloumi cheese, sliced into 4 slabs ½ pound
- basil leaves, torn 5
- finely chopped flat-leaf parsley 2 tablespoons

Nutrition Information
Carbs: 8 g

Proteins: 9 g

Fats: 15 g

Instructions

1. On a medium high flame pre-heat a grill or grill pan.
2. On a serving plate arrange tomatoes. Squeeze lemon lightly over them flavour with pepper and flaky salt.
3. Oil the grill grates with oil and add halloumi and cook, turn once or till marks of grill appear and cheese is thoroughly warmed. It generally takes one minute per side. Moisten salad with olive oil. Dot with parsley and basil. Serve at once.

Harissa Chickpea Stew with Eggplant and Millet

Serving size: 1
Servings per recipe: 4
Calories: 600
Preparation time: 35 minutes
Cooking time: 1 hour

Ingredients:

Lemon Herb Chicken

- boneless, skinless chicken breasts 1½ pounds
- extra-virgin olive oil 3 tablespoons
- Zest and juice of 2 lemons
- chopped fresh oregano 1 tablespoon
- chopped fresh dill 1 tablespoon
- chopped fresh parsley 3 tablespoons
- Kosher salt and freshly ground black pepper as per taste

Salad

- Barley 1 cup
- chicken broth 2½ cups
- Zest and juice of 1 lemon
- whole-grain mustard 1 tablespoon
- dried oregano 1 teaspoon
- extra-virgin olive oil ⅓ cup
- Kosher salt and freshly ground black pepper as per taste
- red-leaf lettuce, chopped 2 heads red onion, halved and
- thinly sliced- 1
- cherry tomatoes, sliced 1 pint
- sliced avocados- 2

Nutrition Information

Lemon Herb Chicken
Carbs: 4 g
Proteins: 39 g
Fats: 15 g

Salad
Carbs: 60 g
Protein: 15 g
Fats: 36 g

Instructions:

1. In a re-sealable plastic bag place the chicken. Whisk olive oil, lemon juice, oregano, parsley, dill and lemon zest in a medium sized bowl. Put this marinade into the bag, seal it and keep in fridge for 30 minutes.
2. Take a medium saucepan, put chicken broth, barley, and bring it to simmer over medium heat. At simmering, cover it and keep cooking till barley is soft, drain water and reserve.
3. Whisk mustard, oregano, lemon zest and juice in a medium bowl. Flavour with pepper and salt.
4. Ready grill for high heat. Take the chicken out from marinade and flavour with pepper and salt.
5. Keep grilling the chicken until properly charred and thoroughly cooked (10-12 minutes), flip in between as required. Take it off the grill and reserve.
6. Toss tomatoes, onion and lettuce in a large bowl. Add dressing, it should be toss well for proper coating.

Five-Minute Heirloom Tomato Toast

Serving size: 2
Servings per recipe: 3
Calories: 177
Preparation time: 5 minutes
Cooking time: 10 minutes

Ingredients:

- small heirloom tomato, diced-1
- Persian cucumber, diced-1
- extra-virgin olive oil 1 teaspoon
- dried oregano Pinch
- Kosher salt and freshly ground black pepper as per taste
- low-fat whipped cream cheese 2 teaspoons Trader Joe's
- Whole Grain Crisp bread 2 pieces
- balsamic glaze 1 teaspoon

Nutrition Information

Carbs: 24 g

Proteins: 3 g

Fats: 8 g

Instructions

1. Combine cucumber, olive oil, tomato and oregano in medium sized bowl. Flavour with salt and pepper.
2. On the bread top apply the cream cheese and top it with mixture of tomato and cucumber as well as the balsamic glaze.

Eggplant and Herb Flatbread

Serving size: 2
Servings per recipe: 8
Calories: 297
Preparation time: 5 minute
Cooking time: 1 hour

Ingredients:

- Eggplants 2 lbs
- Garlic cloves- 6
- ground cumin ¼ teaspoon
- paprika ¼ teaspoon
- olive oil 2 tablespoons
- lemon juice 1 tablespoon
- tahini ¼ cup
- Kosher salt to taste

For the Flatbread

-

- pizza dough 1/2 pound (whole wheat)
- scallions sliced on a hard angle 1 bunch
- mint parsley and basil leaves 1 large handful
- lemon juice 1 tablespoon
- Kosher salt and freshly cracked black pepper to taste
- Olive oil
- feta crumbled ½ cup

Nutrition Information: Carbs: 31 g; **Proteins:** 15 g; **Fats:** 12 g

Instructions

1. With a fork prick the eggplant all over. Under the broil roast them until skin is blackened all over and the eggplant is soft. Keep in a bowl and cover with plastic wrap. Keep aside to cool for around 45 minutes.
2. Remove the skin of eggplant and cut the inside, discard skin and keep in a tidy large bowl.
3. Mince garlic finely, add a little salt while mincing to combine. Put the eggplant. Now add olive oil, cumin, paprika and lemon juice stir to combine. Put tahini budge to combine. Check taste and add salt and lemon juice as required.
4. Pre-heat oven to 450 F.
5. Roll the dough into a rectangle about the size of sheet pan on a light floured surface. Shift to an oiled baking sheet, mizzle with olive oil. Bake till it turns golden. After removing from oven apply a thick layer of eggplant mixture.
6. Combine mint, scallions, parsley, basil and scallions in a small bowl. Toss with salt, pepper and lemon juice. Mizzle with olive oil and toss. Now put mixture of herbs over the layer of eggplant. Give a finishing touch with feta. Serve at once.

5-Minute Mediterranean Couscous with Tuna and Pepperoncini

Serving size: 1
Servings per recipe: 4
Calories: 226
Preparation time: 3 minutes
Cooking time: 12 minutes

Ingredients:

<u>Couscous</u>

- chicken broth or water 1 cup
- couscous 1¼ cups
- kosher salt ¾ teaspoon

<u>Accompaniments</u>

- tuna Two 5-ounce oil packed cans
- cherry tomatoes, halved 1 pint
- sliced pepperoncini ½ cup
- chopped fresh parsley ⅓ cup
- capers ¼ cup
- Extra-virgin olive oil, for serving
- Kosher salt and freshly ground black pepper to taste
- quartered lemon 1

Nutrition Information

Carbs: 44 g

Proteins: 8 g

Fats: 1 g

Instructions

1. Bring water or broth to boil in a small pot on medium flame. Take the pot off the pot, stir the couscous and with a lid cover the pot. Leave for 10 minutes.
2. Toss together tomatoes, tuna, pepperoncini, capers and parsley.
3. With a cork fluff the couscous flavour with pepper and salt, and mizzle with olive oil. With a tuna mixture top the couscous. Your dish is ready to be served with lemon wedges.

Pesto Quinoa Bowls With Roasted Veggies and Labneh

Serving size: 1
Servings per recipe: 4
Calories: 862
Preparation time: 10 minutes
Cooking time: 40 minutes

Ingredients:

- large Japanese eggplant, cubed 1
- medium zucchini, cubed-1
- cherry tomatoes, sliced in half 1 pint
- romano (or green) beans Handful
- Extra-virgin olive oil
- Kosher salt and freshly ground black pepper to taste
- quinoa, rinsed 1 cup
- pesto ½ cup (home-made)
- labneh or Greek yogurt 1 cup
- minced garlic clove- 1
- Juice from ½ lemon
  cilantro or parsley (or both!), roughly chopped Handful
-

Nutrition Information: Carbs: 96 g; **Proteins:** 32 g; **Fats:** 42 g

Instructions

1. Fore-heat oven to 400 ° F. with a parchment paper line large baking sheet. Set up zucchini, eggplant, cherry tomatoes and beans on it. Mizzle olive oil over the vegetables and flavour with pepper and salt. Keep roasting till all the vegetables turn tender or get caramelized. It takes generally 30-40 minutes.
2. Put quinoa to a medium sized saucepan along with 2 cups of water and a little salt. Bring it to boil, with a lid cover it, reduce flame to simmer and cook for around 15 minutes. After quinoa gets cooked, remove the lid, with a fork fluff it and allow it to cool. After quinoa are cooled a bit, using a pesto toss it.
3. In a small bowl mix garlic, lemon juice, herbs and labneh.
4. Set up each bowl by placing quinoa and put up veggies in a row to give rainbow like look. Thereafter add a dollop of labneh on one side.

Greek Yogurt Chicken Salad Stuffed Peppers

Serving size: 1
Servings per recipe: 6
Calories: 116
Preparation time: 30 minutes
Cooking time: 0 minute

Ingredients:

- Greek yogurt ⅔ cup
- Dijon mustard 2 tablespoons
- seasoned rice vinegar 2 tablespoons
- Kosher salt and freshly ground black pepper
- chopped fresh parsley ⅓ cup
- rotisserie chicken, cubed-1
- sliced stalks celery-4
- sliced and divided scallions 1 bunch
- quartered and divided cherry tomatoes, 1 pint
- diced English cucumber, ½
- halved and seeds removed bell peppers- 3

Nutrition Information

Carbs: 16 g

Proteins: 7 g

Fats: 3 g

Instructions

1. Whisk Greek yogurt, mustard and rice vinegar in a medium sized bowl; flavour with pepper and salt. Now stir in parsley.
2. Add celery, chicken and three quarters of tomatoes, scallions and cucumber. Budge well to combine.
3. Among the bell pepper boats divide chicken salad.
4. Dress with remaining tomatoes, scallions and cucumber.

15-Minute Mezze Plate with Toasted Za ' atar Pita Bread

Serving size: 1
Servings per recipe: 4
Calories: 731
Preparation time: 10 minutes
Cooking time: 5 minutes

Ingredients:

- whole-wheat pita rounds 4
- extra-virgin olive oil 4 tablespoons
- za'atar 4 teaspoons
- Greek yogurt 1 cup
- Kosher salt and freshly ground black pepper to taste
- Hummus 1 cup
- marinated artichoke hearts 1 cup
- sliced roasted red peppers 1 cup
- assorted olives 2 cups
- cherry tomatoes 2 cups
- salami 4 ounces

Nutrition Information
Carbs: 62 g
Proteins: 26 g
Fats: 48 g

Instructions

1. Over medium flame heat a large skillet. Each side of pita is to be brushed with olive oil, flavour it with zaátar.
2. Now work in parts, add pita to the skillet and toast till it turns golden brown, for around 2 minutes each side. Cut each pita into quarters.
3. With salt and pepper flavour Greek yogurt.
4. For assembling divide Greek yogurt, artichoke hearts, roasted red, pitas, hummus, tomatoes and salami in four plates.

Greek Lemon Chicken Skewers with Tzatziki Sauce

Serving size: 1
Servings per recipe: 6
Calories: 68
Preparation time: 30 minutes
Cooking time: 1 hour

Ingredients:

TZATZIKI SAUCE

- Greek yogurt 1 cup
- Diced European cucumber- ½
- extra-virgin olive oil 1 tablespoon
- lemon juice 2 tablespoons
- Garlic powder Pinch
- Salt and freshly ground black pepper to taste
- fresh chopped dill ¼ cup

Nutrition Information
Carbs: 3 g
Proteins: 4 g
Fats: 5 g

Instructions

1. Mix yogurt, olive oil, cucumber, lemon juice and garlic powder in a medium sized bowl. Flavour with pepper and salt and then budge in a dill.
2. Whisk yogurt with lemon zest, lemon juice, oregano, and cayenne and garlic powder in a small bowl.
3. Rub the chicken with yogurt-lemon mixture to coat well in a separate bowl.
4. On each skewer put one piece of chicken, weave the strip back and forth while threading it on to the skewer for securing it.
5. With olive oil brush both sides of skewers and then flavour with pepper and salt. In batch cook on fore-heated grill or grill pan, char nicely on both side, for 4-5 minutes on each side.
6. Garnish with tzatziki sauce and parsley. Serve at once.

This Eggplant Pizza is Low-Carb, Gluten-Free and Ready in Under An Hour

Serving Size: 1
Servings per recipe: 6
Calories: 257
Preparation time: 15 minutes
Cooking time: 20 minutes

Ingredients:

- Eggplants-1 large or 2 medium
- olive oil ⅓ cup
- Salt and freshly ground black pepper to taste
- marinara sauce homemade 1¼ cups
- shredded mozzarella cheese 1½ cups
- cherry tomatoes, halved 2 cups
- torn basil leaves ½ cup

Nutrition Information
Carbs: 13 g
Proteins: 8 g
Fats: 20 g

Instructions

1. Fore-heat oven to 400 °F. With a parchment paper line a baking sheet.
2. Knife the ends off the eggplant(s) and then cut into ¾ inch-thick slices. Set up these slices on the readied baking sheets. Brush both sides of the slices with olive oil. Flavour with pepper and salt.
3. Roast slices of eggplant until almost tender (10-12 minutes).
4. Take the trays out from the oven and spread marinara sauce on top of each piece.
5. Place the pizza in the oven roast till the cheese melts and tomatoes get blistered. (5-7 minutes).
6. Garnish pizza with basil and serve hot.

Wild Alaska Salmon and Smashed Cucumber Grain Bowls

Serving size: 1
Servings per recipe: 4
Calories: 841
Preparation time: 15 minutes
Cooking time: 40 minutes

Ingredients:

- Farro 2 cups
- Juice of 2 lemons
- Dijon mustard 2 tablespoons
- minced garlic clove-1
- extra-virgin olive oil ⅓ cup plus 2 tablespoons
- Kosher salt and freshly ground black pepper to taste
- European cucumber, cut into 1-inch chunks 1
- seasoned rice vinegar ¼ cup
- chopped fresh parsley ¼ cup
- chopped fresh mint ¼ cup

  chopped fresh dill ¼ cup
- Four wild Alaska sockeye salmon fillets 6-ounce

Nutrition Information

Carbs: 69 g

Proteins: 49 g

Fats: 43 g

Instructions

1. Large pot of salted water is brought to boil. Put farro into boiling water. Cook until wilted. (25-30 minutes) Drain.
2. In a medium bowl shift farro. Now mix mustard, garlic, lemon juice and 1/3 cup of olive oil; flavour with pepper and salt.
3. Roughly smash cucumber chunks with large fork in a separate medium sized bowl. After adding rice vinegar toss to combine. Flavour with pepper and salt, add mint, dill and parsley.
4. Heat the remaining 2 tablespoon olive oil in a skillet over medium heat. Flavour salmon with salt and pepper. Next ass fillets to hot oil and keep cooking till the desired level of doneness is attained or 8-10 minutes.
5. Now divide farro into four bowls. Break one salmon fillet in each bowl do topping with herbs and cucumbers.

Harissa Potato Salad

Serving size: 1
Servings per recipe: 4
Calories: 231
Preparation time: 10 minutes
Cooking time: 15 minutes

Ingredients:

- 1 1/2 lbs baby potatoes (leave the skins on)
- 2 tablespoons harissa paste
- 6 ounces low-fat or non-fat Greek yogurt
- 1/4 tsp. salt
- 1/4 tsp. pepper
- Juice of 1 lemon
- 1/4 cup finely diced red onion
- 1/4 cup fresh cilantro or parsley, roughly chopped

Nutrition Information
Carbs: 28 g

Proteins: 3 g

Fats: 12 g

Instructions

1. In a big pot place potatoes cover and add 2" of salted cold water. Bring it to boil on medium flame. Keep cooking potatoes until fork tender. (9-11 minutes). Drain water and keep aside to cool a bit.
2. Whisk harissa, salt pepper, Greek Yogurt and lemon juice in a small bowl.
3. Shift the potatoes to a large bowl. Put dressing gently fold it in until potatoes are well coated. Thereafter, fold carefully in herbs and diced red onion
4. Serve at once warm at room temperature or when chilled.

Greek Lemon Chicken Soup

Serving size: 1
Servings per recipe: 4
Calories: 252.8
Preparation time: 10
Cooking time: 20

Ingredients:

- olive oil, divided 2 tablespoons
- boneless, skinless chicken thighs, cut into 1-inch chunks 1 pound
- Kosher salt and freshly ground black pepper to taste
- minced garlic cloves, 4
- diced onion 1
- peeled and diced carrots, 3
- diced stalks celery, 2
- dried thyme 1/2 teaspoon
- chicken stock 8 cups
- bay leaves 2
- cannellini beans, rinsed and drained 15.5 ounce
- baby spinach 4 cups
- freshly squeezed lemon juice, or more, to taste 2
- tablespoons chopped fresh parsley leaves 2 tablespoons
- chopped fresh dill 2 tablespoons

Nutrition Information: Carbs: 30.7 g; **Proteins:** 24.8 g; **Fats:** 4.4 g

Instructions

1. In a large stockpot or Dutch oven heat 1 tablespoon olive oil over medium flame. Flavour chicken thighs with pepper and salt as per your taste. Put chicken in the stockpot, keep cooking until golden (2-3 minutes) keep aside.
2. Now add 1 tablespoon to stockpot. Add onion, carrots, celery and garlic. Keep cooking until soft, keep stirring in between. Budge thyme until aromatic (1 minute).
3. Whisk in bay leaves and chicken stock. Bring to boil; lower heat stir chicken and cannellini beans, budge occasionally, until slightly thick. (10-15 minutes)
4. Now stir spinach to the point of wilting (for 2 minutes). Budge in parsley, dill and lemon juice; flavour with pepper and salt as per your taste. Serve at once.

Mediterranean Bento Lunch

Serving size: 1 Bento box

Servings per recipe: 1

Calories: 497

Preparation time: 5 minute

Cooking time: 15 minute

Ingredients:

- chickpeas, rinsed ¼ cup
- diced cucumber ¼ cup
- diced tomato ¼ cup
- diced olives 1 tablespoon
- crumbled feta cheese 1 tablespoon
- chopped fresh parsley 1 tablespoon
- hummus 2 tablespoons
- extra-virgin olive oil ½ teaspoon
- red-wine vinegar 1 teaspoon
- grilled turkey breast tenderloin or chicken breast 3 ounces
- grapes 1 cup
- whole-wheat pita bread, quartered- 1

Nutrition information

Carbs: 60. 5 g

Proteins: 36.7 g

Fats: 13.8 g

Instructions

1. In a medium bowl toss tomato, cucumber, chickpeas, feta, parsley, oil, olives and vinegar. Pack this in a medium-sized container.
2. In a medium container place turkey or chicken.
3. Pack hummus in a dip-size container and grapes and pita in small containers.

Greek Meatball Mezze Bowls

Serving size: 2 ½ cups

Serving per recipe: 4

Calories: 392

Preparation time: 10 minutes

Cooking time: 35 minutes

Ingredients:

- frozen chopped spinach, thawed 1 cup
- 93%-lean ground turkey 1 pound
- crumbled feta cheese ½ cup
- garlic powder ½ teaspoon
- dried oregano ½ teaspoon
- salt, divided ⅜ teaspoon
- ground pepper, divided ⅜ teaspoon
-

- cooked quinoa, cooled 2 cups
- lemon juice 2 tablespoons
- olive oil 1 tablespoon
- chopped parsley ½ cup
- chopped mint 3 tablespoons
- sliced cucumber 2 cups
- cherry tomatoes 1 pint

tzatziki ¼ cup

Nutrition information

Carbs: 29.3

Protein: 32.4

Fats: 17.2

Instructions

1. First of all squeeze excess moisture from spinach. In a medium bowl by mixing well combine the spinach with turkey, feta, garlic powder, oregano, 1/8 teaspoon salt and 1/8 pepper. Prepare mixture into 12 meatballs. Over medium flame a large non-stick skillet. Coat it with spray. Take the meatball in batches if required now add to the pan and keep cooking until evenly brown and are not pink anymore in the center, it will take 10-12 minutes. Set the meatballs aside to cool.
2. Now in a medium bowl combine quinoa, lemon juice, oil, parsley, mint and the remaining ¼ teaspoon salt and pepper each. Each is to be topped with 3 meatballs, ½ cup cucumbers and ½ cup cherry tomatoes.
3. After this seal the containers and refrigerate for up to 4 days. Now divide tzatziki in 4 small containers and put in the fridge.
4. Before you serve, shift the meatballs to a microwave-safe container and heat until steaming. Come back to original container and serve with tzatzik

Mediterranean Chicken with Orzo Salad

Serving size: 1/2 Chicken Breast & 1 Cup Orzo Salad

Serving per recipe: 4

Calories: 402

Preparation time: 10 minutes

Cooking time: 40 minutes

Ingredients:

- skinless, boneless chicken breasts (8 ounces each), halved-2
- extra-virgin olive oil, divided 3 tablespoons
- lemon zest 1 teaspoon
- salt, divided ½ teaspoon
- ground pepper, divided ½ teaspoon
- whole-wheat orzo ¾ cup
- thinly sliced baby spinach 2 cups
- chopped cucumber 1 cup
- chopped tomato 1 cup
- chopped red onion ¼ cup
- crumbled feta cheese ¼ cup
- chopped Kalamata olives 2 tablespoons
- lemon juice 2 tablespoons
- garlic clove, grated-1
- chopped fresh oregano 2 teaspoons

Nutrition information: Carbs: 28.3 g; Protein: 32 g; Fats: 27.5 g

Instruction:

1. Pre-heat oven to 425 degrees F.
2. First brush chicken with 1 tbsp. oil and sprinkle with lemon zest and ¼ tsp. salt and one tsp. pepper. Put it a baking dish. Keep baking until an instant-read thermometer after insertion shows 165 degrees F, or for 25-30 minutes.
3. By that time, bring 32 ounces of water to boil in a medium saucepan over high flame. After this add orzo and cook for 8 minutes. Now add spinach and cook for another minutes. Drain and wash with cold water. Drain well and shift to a large bowl. Add tomato, cucumber, onion, olives and feta. Stir to combine.
4. In a small bowl whisk the remaining 2 tbsp. Oil, garlic, lemon juice, oregano and the remaining ¼ teaspoon salt and pepper each. Now stir everything except 1 tbsp. of the dressing over the chicken. Serve it with salad.

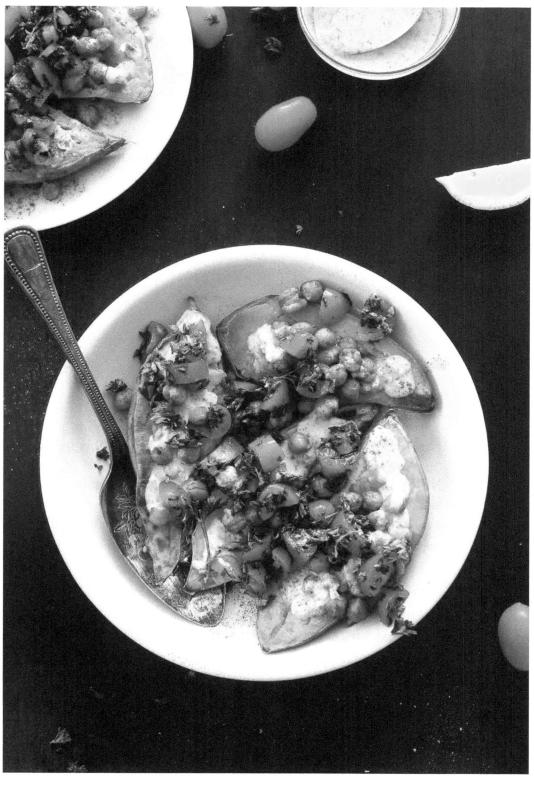

Mediterranean Portobello Mushroom Pizzas with Arugula Salad

Serving size: 1
Servings per recipe: 2
Calories: 264
Preparation time: 10 minutes
Cooking time: 35 minutes

Ingredients:

- large portobello mushroom caps (about 4 oz. each), gills removed 8
- olive oil 2 tablespoons., divided 1 tsp. , divided ground pepper ½
- teaspoon
- pizza or tomato sauce ½ cup
- lightly packed baby spinach, chopped 2 cups sun-
- dried chopped tomatoes ½ cup (about 8) rinsed and
- chopped artichoke hearts, 1 (14 ounce)

Nutrition Information

Carbs: 25 g

Proteins: 14 g

Fats: 13 g

Instructions

4. Fore-heat oven to 400 F°. Use foil to line a large baking sheet and keep it on a wire rack. With 1 tablespoon olive oil brush tops of portobello caps. Now place them undersides-up on the rack. For ten minutes roast. Change side and roast for another 5 minutes.

5. Take out portobellos from the oven and flip them carefully to bring the underside up. Flavour with ¼ teaspoon pepper. Apply 1 tablespoon sauce inside each cap. Divide sun-dried tomatoes, mozzarella and feta among caps. Sprinkle with Italian flavours. Now place portobellos to the oven again and baking to the point when cheese melts and turns brown (10-15 minutes).

6. Whisk the left 1 tablespoon and 1 teaspoon oil and 1/8 teaspoon pepper and lemon juice in a medium sized bowl. Now put arugula and to coat toss.

7. Dress the Portobello pizzas with basil and serve with arugula salad.

Slow-Cooker Mediterranean Quinoa with Arugula

Serving size: 1 ½ cup
Servings per recipe: 6
Calories: 352
Preparation time: 25 minutes
Cooking time: 3-4 hours

Ingredients:

- cups unsalted vegetable stock 2 ¼
- uncooked quinoa, rinsed 1 ½ cups
- sliced red onions (from 1 onion) 1 cup
- minced garlic cloves, 2 (about 2 teaspoons)
- can no-salt-added chickpeas (garbanzo beans), drained and rinsed 1 (15.5 ounce)
- olive oil 2 ½ tablespoons
- kosher salt ¾ teaspoon
- fresh lemon juice (from one lemon) 2 teaspoons
- drained, chopped roasted red bell peppers (from jar) ½ cup
- baby arugula 4 cups (about 4 ounces)
- feta cheese, crumbled 2 ounces (about 1/2 cup)
- kalamata olives, halved lengthwise 12 pitted
- coarsely chopped fresh oregano 2 tablespoons

Nutrition Information
Carbs: 46 g
Proteins: 12 g
Fats: 13 g

Instructions

1. In a 5-6 quart slow cooker stir stock, quinoa, garlic, chickpeas, onions, 1 ½ teaspoons of olive oil and ½ teaspoon of salt. Close the cooker lid and cook on low flame until the quinoa is soft and stock is absorbed (3-4 hours).
2. Turn the slow cooker off. With a fork fluff the quinoa mixture. Now mix lemon juice, remaining 2 tablespoon olive oil and ¼ teaspoon salt with a whisker. Now put the red bell peppers and olive oil into slow cooker. Gently toss to combine and fold in the same manner in the arugula. Keep it this way for 10 minutes or until the arugula is gently wilted. Mizzle each serving evenly with feta cheese, olive oil and oregano.

Walnut-Rosemary Crusted Salmon

Serving size: 3 ounces
Servings per recipe: 4
Calories: 222
Preparation time: 10 minutes
Cooking time: 10 minutes

Ingredients:

- Dijon mustard 2 teaspoons
- minced clove garlic 1
- lemon zest ¼ teaspoon
- lemon juice 1 teaspoon
- chopped fresh rosemary 1 teaspoon
- Honey ½ teaspoon
- kosher salt ½ teaspoon
- crushed red pepper ¼ teaspoon
- panko breadcrumbs 3 tablespoons
- finely chopped walnuts 3 tablespoons
- extra-virgin olive oil 1 teaspoon
- skinless salmon fillet, fresh or frozen 1 (1 pound)
- Olive oil cooking spray 1 serving
- Chopped fresh parsley and lemon wedges for garnish

Nutrition Information
Carbs: 4 g
Proteins: 24 g
Fats: 12 g

Instructions

1. Fore-heat oven to 425 F°. With a parchment paper line a large rimmed baking sheet.
2. In a small bowl combine lemon juice, lemon zest, mustard, rosemary, honey, salt and crushed red pepper. In another small bowl combine panko, walnuts and oil.
3. On the prepared baking sheet place salmon. Over the fish spread mustard mixture and sprinkle with mixture of panko, press to adhere. With cooking spray coat lightly.
4. Bake until fish flakes set easily with a fork (8-12 minutes).
5. Sprinkle with parsley and serve with lemon wedges, if desired.

Mediterranean Stuffed Chicken Breasts

Serving size: ½ breast
Servings per recipe: 8
Calories: 179
Preparation time: 35 minutes
Cooking time: 25 minutes

Ingredients:

- crumbled feta cheese ½ cup
- chopped roasted red bell peppers ½ cup
- chopped fresh spinach ½ cup
- Kalamata olives, pitted and quartered ¼ cup
- chopped fresh basil 1 tablespoon
-
- chopped fresh flat-leaf parsley 1 tablespoon
- minced cloves garlic, 2
- boneless, skinless chicken breasts-4 (8 ounce)
- salt ¼ teaspoon
- ground pepper ½ teaspoon
- extra-virgin olive oil 1 tablespoon lemon juice 1 tablespoon

Nutrition Information
Carbs: 1.9 g
Proteins: 24.4 g
Fats: 7.4 g

Instructions

1. Heat oven beforehand to 400 F, in a medium bowl combine feta, spinach, roasted red peppers, olives, basil, parsley and garlic.

2. To form a pocket cut horizontal slit through the thickest portion of each chicken breast. With 1/3 cup of feta mixture stuff each breast pocket; using wooden picks to secure the pockets. With pepper and salt sprinkle the chicken evenly.

3. In a large oven-safe skillet heat oil over medium flame. Set up stuffed breasts upside down, in the pan, cook until golden, about 2 minutes. Flip the chicken carefully. Shift the pan to the oven. Keep baking until as instant-read thermometer is inserted in the thickest portion of the chicken and shows 165 degrees F (20-25 minutes). Drizzle chicken evenly with lemon juice. Keep in mind that wooden picks from the chicken before serving.

Charred Shrimp & Pesto Buddha Bowls

Serving size: 2 ½ cup
Servings per recipe: 4
Calories: 429
Preparation time: 5 minutes
Cooking time: 20 minutes

Ingredients:

- prepared pesto ⅓ cup
- balsamic vinegar 2 tablespoons
- extra-virgin olive oil 1 tablespoon
- salt ½ teaspoon
- ground pepper ¼ teaspoon
- peeled and deveined large shrimp 1 pound (16-20 count), patted dry
- arugula 4 cups
- cooked quinoa 2 cups
- halved cherry tomatoes 1 cup
- diced avocado-1

Nutrition Information
Carbs: 29.3 g
Proteins: 30.9 g
Fats: 22 g

Instructions

1. In a large bowl whisk vinegar, pesto, oil, pepper and salt. Shift 4 tablespoons of mixture. Keep both bowls aside.
2. Over medium flame heat a large cast-iron skillet. Put shrimp and cook stirring till the shrimp gets cooked through and is slightly charred (4-5 minutes) transfer to plate.
3. In a large bowl add quinoa and arugula with vinaigrette and toss to coat. Divide the arugula mixture between 4 bowls. Do topping with tomatoes, avocado and shrimp. Mizzle each bowl with 1 tablespoon of the reserved pesto mixture.

Sheet-Pan Salmon with Sweet Potatoes & Broccoli

Serving size: 2
Servings per recipe: 4
Calories: 504
Preparation time: 15 minutes
Cooking time: 20 minutes

Ingredients:

- 3 tablespoons low-fat mayonnaise
- 1 teaspoon chili powder
- 2 medium sweet potatoes, peeled and cut into 1-inch cubes
- 4 teaspoons olive oil, divided
- ½ teaspoon salt, divided
- ¼ teaspoon ground pepper, divided
- 4 cups broccoli florets (8 oz.; 1 medium crown)
- 1 ¼ pounds salmon fillet, cut into 4 portions
- 2 limes, 1 zested and juiced, 1 cut into wedges for serving ¼
- cup crumbled feta or cotija cheese ½ cup chopped fresh
- cilantro

Nutrition Information: Carbs: 34 g; Proteins: 34 g; Fats: 26 g

Instructions

1. Fore-heat the oven to 425 degrees F. With a foil line a large rimmed baking sheet and coat with cooking spray.
2. Combine chilli powder and mayonnaise in a small bowl. Keep aside.
3. In a medium bowl toss sweet potatoes with 2 teaspoon oil, ¼ teaspoon salt and 1/8 teaspoon pepper. Spread it on the baking sheet prepared. For 15 minutes roast it.
4. In the same bowl toss broccoli with the remaining 2 teaspoon oil, 1/8 teaspoon pepper ¼ salt. Now remove the baking sheet form the oven. Now stir the sweet potatoes and push them to the sides of the pan. Move salmon in the center of the pan and on either side spread broccoli, among sweet potatoes. Spread 2 tablespoons of mayonnaise mixture over the salmon. Bake for around 15 minutes or until the sweet potatoes are tender and salmon flakes conveniently with a fork.
5. By that time, add lime zest and lemon juice to remaining 1 tablespoon low fat mayonnaise; mix it well.
6. Among 4 plates divide salmon and top with cheese and cilantro. Divide the broccoli and the sweet potatoes among the plates mizzle with the lime-mayonnaise sauce. You can serve with wedges of lime and any leftover sauce.

Greek Cauliflower Rice Bowls with Grilled Chicken

Serving size: 4
Servings per recipe: 2
Calories: 411
Preparation time: 5 minutes
Cooking time: 30 minutes

Ingredients:

- extra-virgin olive oil, divided 6 tablespoons plus 1 teaspoon
- cauliflower rice 4 cups
- chopped red onion ⅓ cup
- salt, divided ¾ teaspoon
- chopped fresh dill, divided ½ cup
- boneless, skinless chicken breasts 1 pound
- ground pepper, divided ½ teaspoon
- 3 tablespoons lemon juice
- dried oregano 1 teaspoon
- halved cherry tomatoes 1 cup
- chopped cucumber 1 cup
- 2 tablespoons chopped Kalamata olives
- 2 tablespoons crumbled feta cheese
- 4 wedges Lemon wedges for serving

Nutrition Information: Carbs: 29 g; Proteins: 9.5 g; Fats: 27 g

Instructions

1. Fore-heat grill to medium
2. Over medium high flame heat 2 tablespoon oil in a large skillet. Cook for about 5 minutes or until the cauliflower is softened, stir occasionally. Remove from heat and dodge in ¼ cup dill.
3. Rub 1 teaspoon oil all over chicken. Sprinkle ¼ teaspoon pepper and ¼ teaspoon salt. Flip and grill, check using an instant-read thermometer into the thickest part of the breast. It should show temperature of 165 degrees (15 minutes total) cut in crosswise slices.
4. In a small bowl whisk remaining 4 tablespoons oil, lemon juice, oregano and the ¼ teaspoon salt and pepper.
5. Do part cauliflower rice in four bowls. Top with tomatoes, cucumber, chicken, olives and feta. Sprinkle remaining ¼ cup dill. Mizzle vinaigrette. You can serve with lemon wedges.

Prosciutto Pizza with Corn & Arugula

Serving size: ¼ pizza
Servings per recipe: 4
Calories: 436
Preparation time: 10 minutes
Cooking time: 20 minutes
Ingredients:

- pizza dough, preferably whole-wheat 1 pound
- extra-virgin olive oil, divided 2 tablespoons
- minced clove garlic, 1
- part-skim shredded mozzarella cheese 1 cup
- fresh corn kernels 1 cup
- very thinly sliced prosciutto, torn into 1-inch pieces 1 ounce
- arugula 1 ½ cups
- torn fresh basil ½ cup
- ground pepper ¼ teaspoon

Nutrition Information (per serving)
Carbs: 53.1 g

Proteins: 18.3 g

Fats: 19.9 g

Instructions

1. Fore-heat grill to medium-high flame.

2. On a lightly floured surface roll dough into a 12" oval. Shift it to a lightly floured baking sheet. In a small bowl combine 1 tablespoon oil and garlic. Bring the garlic oil, cheese, dough, corn and prosciutto to the grill.

3. Apply oil on the grill rack. Shift the crust to the grill. Keep grilling the dough until it gets puffed and turn slightly brown (1-2 minutes).

4. Turn the crust over and apply garlic oil on it. top with corn, cheese and prosciutto. Grill, covering it, unit the cheese is melted and the crust is lightly brown at bottom or 2-3 minutes more. Put the pizza back on the baking sheet.

5. Do topping of the pizza with basil, arugula, basil and pepper. Mizzle with the leftover tablespoon oil.

Vegan Mediterranean Lentil Soup

Serving size: 1 cup
Servings per recipe: 6
Calories: 272
Preparation time: 20 minutes
Cooking time: 40 minutes

Ingredients:

- extra-virgin olive oil 2 tablespoons
- chopped yellow onions 1 ½ cups
- chopped carrots 1 cup
- minced garlic, 3 cloves
- no-salt-added tomato paste 2 tablespoons
- reduced-sodium vegetable broth 4 cups
- Water 1 cup
- no-salt-added cannellini beans, rinsed- 1 (15 ounce)
- mixed dry lentils (brown, green and black) 1 cup
- chopped sun-dried tomatoes in oil, drained ½ cup
- Salt ¾ teaspoon
- ground pepper ½ teaspoon
- chopped fresh dill, plus more for garnish 1 tablespoon
- red-wine vinegar 1 ½ teaspoons

Nutrition Information
Carbs: 42 g
Proteins: 13 g
Fats: 7 g

Instructions

1. In a large heavy pot heat oil on medium flame. Add carrots and onion; cook stirring in between, until soft (3-4 minutes). Next add garlic and cook stirring constantly, until mixture is coated evenly, about 1 minutes.

2. Stir in broth, water, cannellini beans, lentils, sun-dried tomatoes, salt and pepper. Bring to a boil over medium-high heat; reduce heat to medium-low. After covering let it summer until lentil turn soft 30-40 minutes.

3. Take off from flame and stir in vinegar and dill. You can add additional dill as per your taste.

BBQ Shrimp with Garlicky Kale & Parmesan-Herb Couscous

Serving size: 3 Oz. Shrimp, 1 Cup Kale & 1/2 Cup Couscous Each
Servings per recipe: 4
Calories: 414
Preparation time: 10 minutes
Cooking time: 20 minutes

Ingredients:

- low-sodium chicken broth 1 cup
- poultry seasoning ¼ teaspoon
- whole-wheat couscous ⅔ cup
- grated Parmesan cheese ⅓ cup
- butter 1 tablespoon
  extra-virgin olive oil, divided 3
- tablespoons
- chopped kale 8 cups

- water ¼ cup
- smashed garlic clove 1 large
- crushed red pepper ¼ teaspoon
- salt ¼ teaspoon
  peeled and deveined raw shrimp 1
- pound (26-30 per pound)
  barbecue sauce ¼ cup

Nutrition Information: Carbs: 36.4 g; **Proteins:** 32.4 g; **Fats:** 16.9 g

Instructions

1.   In a medium size saucepan combine broth and poultry over medium heat. Bring to boil, stir in couscous. Take off from flame and cover the pan leave it for around 5 minutes. With a fork fluff, then stir in Parmesan and butter. Keep it covered so that it stays warm longer.

2.   In a large skillet heat 1 tablespoon oil on medium heat. Add kale and cook for 1-2 minutes or cook until it looks bright green. Now pour water cover the skillet and cook, stirring until kale is soft for about 3 minutes. Bring heat down to medium low. Dig in the center of kale and add 1 tbps. Oil, garlic and crushed red pepper; cook, constantly for 15 seconds, thereafter, stir the garlic oil into kale and flavour with salt. Shift to a bowl and cover to keep it warm.

Now put tablespoon oil and shrimp to pan. Keep cooking stirring in between until the shrimp are curled and pink (2 minutes) take off from the flame and stir in barbecue sauce. Serve the shrimp with couscous and kale.

Green Shakshuka with Spinach, Chard & Feta

Serving size: 1 Egg & 1/2 Cup Greens
Servings per recipe: 6
Calories: 296
Preparation time: 10 minutes
Cooking time: 20 minutes

Ingredients:

- extra-virgin olive oil ⅓ cup
- finely chopped large onion, 1
- chard, stemmed and chopped 12 ounces
- mature spinach, stemmed and chopped 12 ounces
- dry white wine ½ cup
- small jalapeño or serrano pepper, thinly sliced 1
- cloves garlic, very thinly sliced 2 medium
- kosher salt ¼ teaspoon
- ground pepper ¼ teaspoon low-sodium no-
- chicken or chicken broth ½ cup unsalted butter 2
- tablespoons large eggs- 6
-
- crumbled feta or goat cheese ½ cup

Nutrition Information
Carbs: 8.5 g
Proteins: 10.7 g
Fats: 23.4 g

Instructions

1. In a large skillet heat oil over medium flame. Cook for 7-8 minutes adding onion, stirring in between, until soft and translucent but not brown. Put spinach and chard a few handfuls at a time and cook stirring often until soft. Add wine garlic, jalapeno, garlic, pepper and salt; cook stirring in between to the point wine gets absorbed and the garlic turns wilt. Put butter and broth, cook stirring to the point when butter melts and liquid gets absorbed, 1 to 2 minutes.
2. Crack the eggs over the veggies. Cover the skillet and cook over medium-low flame till the whites are set (3-5 minutes). Take off from flame and dredge with cheese, cover and leave for 2 minutes then serve.

One-Skillet Salmon with Fennel & Sun-Dried Tomato Couscous

Serving size: 4 Oz. Salmon & 1 1/4 Cups Couscous
Servings per recipe: 4
Calories: 543
Preparation time: 10 minutes
Cooking time: 30 minutes

Ingredients:

- Lemon 1

- salmon skinned and cut into 4 portions1 ¼ pounds salt ¼ teaspoon

- ground pepper ¼ teaspoon sun-dried tomato pesto, divided 4 tablespoons extra-virgin olive oil, divided 2 tablespoons

- fennel bulbs, cut into 1/2-inch wedges; fronds reserved 2 medium Israeli

- couscous, preferably whole-wheat 1 cup scallions, sliced- 3

- low-sodium chicken broth1 ½ cups

- sliced green olives ¼ cup

- tablespoons toasted pine nuts

- cloves garlic, sliced

Nutrition Information: Carbs: 46 g: **Proteins:** 38.3 g; **Fats:** 7.6 g

Instructions

1. Grate lemon zest and preserve it. Knife 8 slices of lemon. Flavour lemon with pepper and salt. Next apply 1 ½ tsps. Of pesto on each piece.

2. In a large skillet heat 1 tbs. oil over medium flame. For 2-3 minutes cook half the fennel till it turns brown at the bottom. Turn the flame down and repeat with one tbs. oil and fennel. Shift to the plate. In the pan add scallions and couscous, cook stirring frequently, till the couscous turns lightly toasted (1-2 minutes). Stir in broth, pine nuts, olives, garlic, the reserved zest and the leftover two tablespoons of pesto.

3. Take the couscous and nestle fennel and salmon into it. Using lemon slices top the salmon. Turn down the flame to medium low, cook keeping the pan covered till the salmon is thoroughly cooked (10-15 minutes). Dress with fennel fronds, if you wish to do so.

Chicken & Spinach Skillet Pasta with Lemon & Parmesan

Serving size: Scant 2 Cups
Servings per recipe: 4
Calories: 335
Preparation time: 10 minutes
Cooking time: 25 minutes

Ingredients:

- gluten-free whole-wheat penne pasta 8 ounces
- extra-virgin olive oil 2 tablespoons
- boneless, skinless chicken breast or thighs, trimmed, if necessary, and cut into bite-size pieces 1 pound
- salt ½ teaspoon
- ground pepper ¼ teaspoon
- garlic, minced 4 cloves
- dry white wine ½ cup
- Juice and zest of 1 lemon
- chopped fresh spinach 10 cups
- grated Parmesan cheese, divided 4 tablespoons

Nutrition Information

Carbs: 24.9 g

Proteins: 28.7 g

Fats: 12.3 g

Instructions

1. Follow cooking directions given on package to cook pasta.
2. In a large high-sided skillet heat oil. By that time, put chicken, add pepper and salt, cook, stirring now and then, just cook through for 5-7 minutes. Now add garlic cook till aromatic for about 1 minute. Stir in lemon juice, wine, lemon juice and zest. Now bring it to simmer.
3. Remove from flame. Stir in spinach and cooked pasta. Cover the skillet and leave it until the spinach is soft. Divide it in four plate and add toppings over each with 1 tablespoon of Parmesan.

Baked chicken and Ricotta Meatballs

Serving size: 5 balls
Servings per recipe: 4
Calories: 454
Preparation time: 15 minutes
Cooking time: 20 minutes

Ingredients:

- broccolini, rough stems trimmed and thick pieces cut lengthwise 14 ounces (400g)
- ends trimmed and thinly sliced lemon, 1
- extra-virgin olive oil, divided 4 tablespoons Kosher salt
- and freshly ground black pepper to taste crushed red
- pepper flakes, or more if desired ½ teaspoon large egg 1
- grated garlic cloves, 2
- ricotta cheese, drained and lightly salted ¾ cup
- parsley leaves and fine stems, roughly chopped ½
- cup panko breadcrumbs ¾ cup
- ground chicken, preferably dark meat 1 pound
- Juice of 1 lemon
- Grated Parmesan, for sprinkling (optional)

Nutrition Information: Carbs: 20 g; **Proteins:** 36 g; **Fats:** 27 g

Instructions

1. Fore-heat the oven at 425°F

2. Toss the broccoli, lemon slices with 3 tablespoons of the olive oil, salt, red pepper flakes and pepper on a baking sheet. Apply evenly on the baking sheet and keep aside while meatballs are made.

3. Beat the egg, thereafter add the garlic, ricotta, 1 tsp. salt, pepper, parsley and rest of the oil, breadcrumbs and meat, and use with your hands in order to combine it gently (if you do too much mushing will make these items dry and tough.) the pieces of meat should be visible through seasoning. Wet your lightly with water and oil and roll the meat into 20 loose round shaped, a little smaller than golf

balls, use a smaller rolling motion between your hands. The water you used will keep them sticking to your hands. Place large pieces of baking parchment on the counter to make it easy for you to clean.

4. On the baking sheet nestle the meatballs between the broccoli and lemon. Keep baking until the meatballs are brown and get cooked through and the broccoli becomes crispy. It generally takes 15-20 minutes. Shake the baking sheet to move the meatballs and turn the tray around midway to make sure that it gets evenly cooked.

5. Take it out of the oven, squeeze the lemon juice on top and place it doing division across plates. Give a finishing touch with grated parmesan, if you are using the one.

Chickpea Vegetable Coconut Curry

Serving size: 1
Servings per recipe: 4
Calories: 665
Preparation time: 10 minutes
Cooking time: 20 minutes

Ingredients:

- extra-virgin olive oil1- tablespoon
- thinly sliced red onion-1
- thinly sliced red bell pepper1
- minced fresh ginger, 1 tablespoon
- minced garlic cloves 3
- small head cauliflower, cut into bite-size florets1
- chili powder 2 teaspoons
- ground coriander 1 teaspoon
- red curry paste 3 tablespoons
- coconut milk 14-ounce
- halved lime 1
- chickpeas 28-ounce
- frozen peas 1½ cups
- Kosher salt and freshly ground black pepper to taste
- Steamed rice, for serving (optional)
- chopped fresh cilantro ¼ cup
- thinly sliced scallions-4

Nutrition Information; Carbs: 80 g; **Proteins** 26 g; **Fats:** 31 g

Instructions

1. Heat oil over medium flame in a large saucepan. Add onion and bell pepper, sauté till almost tender, for about 5 minutes. Next add garlic and ginger, sauté until aromatic for around 1 minute.
2. Put cauliflower, toss well so as to combine. Stir in coriander, chili powder, coriander and red curry paste, cook till starts becoming caramelised. It generally takes about a minute.

3. Add coconut milk with a stir and bring it to a simmer on medium low flame. Saucepan should be covered while you continue to simmer until the cauliflower is wilted. It will take 8-10 minutes.

4. Take off the lid and squeeze lemon juice into the curry, stir it well to combine. Now add chickpeas, peas, flavour with pepper and salt. Next bring it back to simmer.

5. It is recommended to serve it with rice and dressing should be done of each portion with a tablespoon of cilantro and 1 tablespoon scallion.

Broccoli Rabe and Burrata with Lemon

Serving size: 1

Servings per recipe: 4

Calories: 198

Preparation time: 2 minutes

Cooking time: 8 minutes

Ingredients:

- broccoli rabe, tips of stems trimmed off 1 bunch
- extra-virgin olive oil, plus more for drizzling 1 to 2 tablespoons
- sliced garlic cloves, 2
- red-pepper flakes ¼ teaspoon
- burrata or fresh mozzarella 4 ounces
- fresh lemon juice ½ tablespoon
- crushed, toasted pistachios 2 tablespoons
- Flaky sea salt, for serving

Nutrition
Carbs: 6 g

Proteins: 11 g

Fats: 15 g

Instructions:

1. In a large pot bring salted water to boil. For 3 minutes boil the broccoli rabe, thereafter, drain.
2. Heat 1-2 tablespoons of olive oil in a large deep skillet over medium heat. It should cover the bottom of the pan nicely. First stir in garlic and cook for 30 seconds, thereafter stir in red-pepper flakes.
3. In the pan add the broccoli and sauté, shaking the pan and gently toss it so that cooking gets done, until tender (specially the stems), 3-5 minutes.
4. Take off the broccoli rabe from pan and drain off any excess liquid. On a plate arrange broccoli. Tear the burrata and scatter its pieces among the broccoli rabe. Sparge lemon juice, pistachios and salt. Mizzle with olive oil, if you wish to. Your dish is ready to be served.

Tomato Poached Cod with Special Herbs

Serving size: 1 bowl

Servings per recipe: 4

Calories: 261

Preparation time: 5 minutes

Cooking time: 25 minutes

Ingredients:

- extra-virgin olive oil 2 tablespoons
- thinly sliced shallot, 1
- Kosher salt and freshly ground black pepper to taste
- thinly sliced garlic clove, 1
- crushed red pepper flakes, or more, as desired ½ teaspoon
- crushed tomatoes and their liquid 14-ounce
- low-sodium vegetable stock (or water) 1 cup
- cod fillets Four 5-ounce
- parsley or basil leaves and fine stems, roughly chopped or torn, for sprinkling 1 cup
- Toasted crusty bread, for serving

Nutrition; Carbs: 19 g; Proteins: 30 g; Fats: 8 g

Instructions:

1. In a wide shallow skillet heat oil, till it is shimmering. Add salt and shallot, keep stirring until these get soft. Generally it takes 3 minutes. Add pepper and garlic flakes, keep stirring until aromatic, for about 30 seconds more. Pour in stock and tomatoes and turn the flame high and bring the mixture to boil. Turn the flame down to simmer, keep stirring in between, flavour with salt and pepper. Allow it to cook till tomatoes till liquid slightly. It generally takes 8-10 minutes.

2. Flavour the fish with salt and pepper and put the sauce, adjust the heat to maintain a gentle simmer. Cook and spoon the sauce over fillets occasionally, till the fish is covered. Flakes easily when touched, for about 5 minutes. If these don't submerge fully, turn them over halfway. It may take a little longer to cook thick fillet.

3. Between the serving bowls divide the fish and with a spoon put sauce on the top. Give a finishing touch with pepper and parsley and it should be served with bread for dipping.

Chickpea Shawarma Salad

Serving size: 1 dish
Servings per recipe: 2
Calories: 435
Preparation time: 10 minutes
Cooking time: 20 minutes

Ingredients:

CHICKPEAS
- chickpeas 1. 15-ounce (rinsed, drained and dried in a clean towel)
- olive oil 1 Tablespoon
- cumin 1 heaping teaspoon
- smoked paprika 1/2 heaping teaspoon
- turmeric 1/2 heaping teaspoon
- sea salt 1/2 scant teaspoon
- ground cinnamon 1/2 teaspoon
- ground ginger 1/4 teaspoon
- each black pepper, ground coriander + cardamom 1 pinch

SALAD
- spring mix lettuce 5 ounces (organic when possible)
- cherry tomatoes 10 (chopped // organic when possible)
- red onion 1/4 cup (thinly sliced)
- fresh parsley 3/4 cup
- pita chips 20 (slightly crushed // store-bought or homemade* // gluten-free if GF, or sub gluten-free crackers or cooked quinoa)

DRESSING
- hummus 1/2 cup (**DIY** or store-bought)
- garlic 3 cloves (3 cloves yield ~ 1 1/2 Tablespoon // finely minced or grated)
- dried dill 1 teaspoon (or sub 2 teaspoon fresh dill per 1 teaspoon dried)
- medium lemon, juiced 1 (1 lemon yields ~2 Tablespoon or 30 ml)
- Water (to thin)

Nutrition
- ✓ Carbs: 53.3 g
- ✓ Proteins: 19.3 g
- ✓ Fats: 17.3 g

Instructions

1. Heat oven beforehand 400 degrees F. place a rack in the middle of the oven.

2. To a mixing bowl add washed and dried chickpeas. Put olive oil and flavours, toss mixture to combine. Lightly mash half the chickpeas (leaving the other half whole) with a fork to help them cook faster and sprinkle seasoning more easily.

3. Taste a chickpea and adjust flavour as required. Thereafter set a single layer on a bare baking sheet and bake for 20-22 minutes, or until golden brown and crispy. Then set aside.

4. By that time, do preparation for salad ingredients and to a bowl. Reserve pita chips for later. Keep it aside.

5. For preparing the dressing, add hummus, garlic, dill, and lemon juice to a small mixing bowl and using a whisk to combine it. Thereafter add warm water and keep whisking until pourable.

6. When you want to serve add baked chickpeas and pita chips to the salad and half of dressing. Toss in order to combine.

7. Put in the serving dishes and serve with the remaining dressing items.

8. If you want to have best result, store leftovers separately. It stays for 2-3 days, though best when fresh.

Mediterranean Diet Snacks Recipes

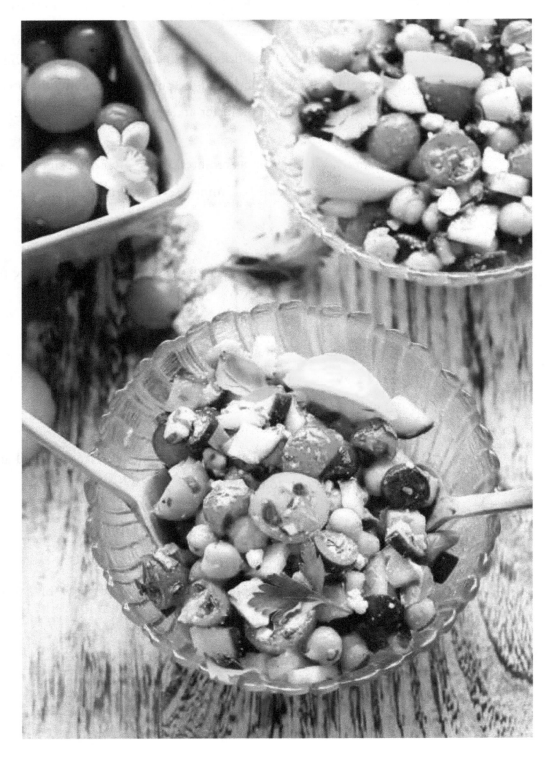

Minute Mediterranean Chickpea Salad

Serving size: 1
Servings per recipe: 4
Calories: 196
Preparation time: 15 minutes
Cooking time: 0 minute

Ingredients:

- Chickpeas 1.15 oz (drained, rinsed and loose shells removed)
- cherry tomatoes halved 1 pint
- finely chopped cucumber 1/2
- sliced black olives 1/4 cup
- herbed feta or plain 1/4 cup
- Juice of 1 lemon
- extra virgin olive oil 2 tbsp
- red wine vinegar 1 tbsp
- fresh parsley finely chopped 1/4 cup
- fresh basil finely chopped 3 tbsp
- garlic powder 1/4 tsp
- Pinch of sea salt and black pepper

Nutrition Information

Carbs: 22g

Proteins: 7 g

Fats: 11 g

Instructions

1. Everything is to be combined in a large bowl, toss well to combine. Your dish is ready to be served.

Lemon Herb Mediterranean Pasta Salad

Serving size: 1
Servings per recipe: 10 g
Calories: 108
Preparation time: 10 minutes
Cooking time: 15 minutes

Ingredients: 12 ounces | 350 grams dry pasta (Penne)

FOR LEMON HERB DRESSING:

- olive oil 1/3 cup
- fresh squeezed lemon juice 2 tablespoons
- red wine vinegar 2 tablespoons
- water 2 tablespoons
- finely chopped fresh parsley 2 tablespoons
- minced garlic , 2 teaspoons
- minced dried oregano , 2 teaspoons
- dried basil 1 teaspoon
- salt 1/2 teaspoon
- Cracked pepper , to taste

FOR SALAD:

- Romaine (or cos) lettuce leaves, washed and dried 4 cups
- large cucumber , diced 1
- avocado , peeled, pitted and chopped 1
- large red pepper (or capsicum), deseeded and cut into thin strips 1/2
- grape or cherry tomatoes, halved 9 ounces (250 grams)
- thinly sliced a red onion , 1/2
- pitted kalamata olives , sliced ½ cup
- sun-dried tomatoes packed in oil , drained 1/3 cup
- crumbled feta cheese 5-6 tablespoons

Nutrition Information: Carbs: 3 g; Proteins: 10 g; Fats: 17.1 g

Instructions

1. In a large pot of salted water boil pasta. Drain in a strainer or colander, thereafter wash under cold water in order to take the heat out. Shift the pasta to a large mixing bowl.
2. When pasta is boiling during that time prepare your dressing. In a large jug whisk together all of the dressing/marinade ingredients.
3. In a salad bowl add all the salad ingredients and pasta, and mizzle with a dressing. All the ingredients should be tossed together till everything is coated evenly in dressing. Season with extra pepper and salt, if you feel like doing it.
4. Serve at once.

Hummus

Serving size: 1 small bowl
Servings per recipe: 8
Calories: 173 kcal
Preparation time: 12 minutes
Cooking time: 8 minutes

Ingredients:

- garlic cloves unpeeled-2
- chickpeas 2 cups (342 g)
- lemon juice ¼ cup (60 ml)
- tahini ⅓ cup (67 g)
- kosher salt ½ teaspoon
- extra-virgin olive oil plus more for drizzling ¼ cup (60 ml)
- paprika for garnish

Nutrition Information
Carbs: 12 g
Proteins: 4 g
Fats: 13 g

Instructions

1. Take a small skillet and heat it over medium heat. Toast garlic to the point of it getting brown, shake pan in between. Peel garlic and set it aside.
2. Now drain the chickpeas, reserve ¼ cup of liquid.
3. Wash the chickpeas under cool water. Remove the outer skin using fingertips. If you feel like you can keep the skin but it may affect the smoothness of your hummus repeatedly.
4. Add ¼ cup of reserved chickpea liquid, tahini and lemon juice in a blender or a food processor.
5. Now process it on high speed for a minute, until it becomes frothy.
6. Add garlic cloves, chickpeas, olive oil and salt.
7. On high speed process for a minute. Scrape the sides down.
8. Next process on high speed till it becomes smooth. It will take about two minutes.
9. Check taste of the hummus. Flavour with more salt if you feel the need.
10. Serve without delay. Mizzle with olive oil and sprinkle with paprika.

Mini Greek Pita Pizzas

Serving size: 1 ½ round
Servings per recipe: 12
Calories: 69 kcal
Preparation time: 10 minutes
Cooking time: 15 minutes

Ingredients:

- whole wheat mini pitas or slide buns divided in half 6
- olive oil 1 tbsp.
- homemade or store-bought hummus 1/4 cup
- chopped tomato seeded 1/3 cup
- chopped cucumber 1/3 cup
- chopped kalamata olives 3 tbsp.
- finely chopped red onion 3 tbsp.
- crumbled feta cheese 2 tbsp.

Nutrition Information

Carbs: 9 g

Proteins: 2 g

Fats: 3 g

Instructions

1. Fore-heat oven to 350 degrees F.
2. Split 6 mini whole-wheat pitas or mini slider buns in half, so as to have 12 small rounds. Now place these rounds on a baking sheet.
3. Apply some oil over each pita with a brush.
4. Now put in the oven and bake for 15 minutes or till these are crispy and lightly brown.
5. Take it out from the oven and apply a thin layer of hummus over each round, going right up to the edge.
6. On each top place equal amount of tomato, cucumber, red onion, olives and feta. Serve without delay.

Healthy Avocado Cilantro White Bean Dip

Serving size: 2 cups dip with 2 heaping tablespoon serving
Servings per recipe: 6
Calories: 144 kcal
Preparation time: 10
Cooking time: 0

Ingredients:

- Organics cannellini beans (approx. 15 oz)
- large ripe avocado-1
- sour cream 2 tablespoon
- jalapeno slices 2 tablespoons
- garlic cloves-2
- Fresh spinach 1/2 cup (just grab a handful!)
- fresh lime juice 2-3 tablespoon
- fresh cilantro plus extra to taste 2 tablespoon
- olive oil plus extra to garnish 2 tablespoon
- ground cumin ½ teaspoon
- salt 1/4 teaspoon

Nutrition Information
Carbs: 18 g
Proteins: 6 g
Fats: 5 g

Instructions

1. In a large food processor place all dip ingredients. Keep processing until smooth.
2. It can be served at once or can be covered and refrigerated until ready to use.
3. You can garnish with sliced cherry tomatoes, cilantro and red onions.
4. Serve with veggies, *O* Organics blue Corn Tortilla chips with flax seed, *O* organics Pita crackers.

Homemade Granola Bars Recipe (Gluten-Free, Vegan, Dairy-Free)

Serving size: 1
Servings per recipe: 12 bars
Calories: 209
Preparation time: 5 minutes
Cooking time: 1 hour 15 minutes

Ingredients:

- Dried Mulberries, chopped 1/3 cup
- Dried Strawberries, chopped 1/3 cup
- Raw Cashews, chopped 1/2 cup
- Organic Peanut Butter 1/2 cup
- large ripe bananas, mashed 2
- Raw Sunflower Seeds 1/3 cup
- Organic Hemp Protein Powder 2 tablespoon
- Gluten Free Rolled Oats 1 cup
- °Organic Flaxseed Meal 2 tablespoon

Nutrition Information
Carbs: 20.5 g
Proteins: 8.0 g
Fats: 11.6 g

Instructions

1. Heat oven beforehand to 350 F. Use a parchment paper and line an 8X8 square baking pan.
2. Combine the peanut butter and mashed banana in a medium mixing bowl using a manual mixer or an electric whisk.
3. Now add rest of the ingredients in the bowl. Using a spatula mix the ingredients until these are well combined and homogeneous mixture becomes obtainable. Shift the mixture to the ready baking pan. Press it down with a spatula till it is uniform and flat on all sides.
4. Bake it for around 25-30 minutes. Allow the granola to get cool for minimum 40-45 minutes prior to removing it from pam and cutting into bars. Bars should be wrapped in wax paper and stored in the fridge in an airtight container for up to one week.

Charcuterie Bistro Lunch Box

Serving size: 1 box
Servings per recipe: 1
Calories: 452
Preparation time: 5 minutes
Cooking time: 0 minute

Ingredients:

- prosciutto slice 1

- halved mozzarella stick 1

- halved breadsticks 2

- dates 2

- grapes ½ cup

- large radishes, 2

- halved or 4 slices English cucumber (1/4-inch)

Nutrition Information
- ✓ **Carbs: 64.7 g**
- ✓ **Proteins: 16.9 g**
- ✓ **Fats: 17.1 g**

Instructions
1. Knife prosciutto in half-length wise, thereafter wrap a slice around each portion of cheese, dates, breadsticks, grapes and radishes (or cucumber) in a sealable container which has 4-cup division. Refrigerate till ready to eat.

Hummus, Feta & Bell Pepper Cracker

Serving size: I crisp bread with topping
Servings per recipe: 1
Calories: 136
Preparation time: 10 minutes
Cooking time: 0 minutes

Ingredients:

- Hummus 2 tablespoons

- large crisp bread, 1 (Whole Grain Crisp bread)

- crumbled feta cheese 2 tablespoons

- diced bell pepper 2 tablespoons

Nutrition Information
- ✓ **Carbs: 13.1**
- ✓ **Proteins: 6 g**
- ✓ **Fats: 7.1 g**

Instructions

1. On crisp bread spread hummus. Do topping with cheese and bell pepper.

Tomato-Basil Skewers

Serving size: 1 skewer
Servings per recipe: 16
Calories: 46
Preparation time: 10 minutes
Cooking time: 0

Ingredients:

- small fresh mozzarella balls 16

- fresh basil leaves 16

- cherry tomatoes 16

- Extra-virgin olive oil, to drizzle 1 teaspoon

- Coarse salt & freshly ground pepper 1/ to taste

Nutrition Information
✓ **Carbs: 1 g**
✓ **Proteins: 2.8**
✓ **Fats: 3.3**

Instructions

1. On a small skewers mozzarella, basil and tomatoes.
2. Mizzle with oil and sprinkle with pepper and salt.

Marinated Olives & Feta

Serving size: 2 tablespoons
Servings per recipe: 12
Calories: 73
Preparation time: 10 minutes
Cooking time: 1 hour 10 minutes

Ingredients:

- sliced pitted olives, such as Kalamata or mixed Greek 1 cup

- diced feta cheese, preferably reduced-fat ½ cup extra-virgin

- olive oil 2 tablespoons and juice of 1 lemon 1 Zest

- , sliced cloves garlic-2

- chopped fresh rosemary 1 teaspoon

- crushed red pepper 1 pinch

- Freshly ground pepper to taste

Nutrition Information
- ✓ **Carbs:** 2 g
- ✓ **Proteins:** 1.1 g
- ✓ **Fats:** 6.8 g

Instructions

1. In a medium bowl combine feta, olives, oil, lemon juice, zest, garlic, rosemary, crushed red pepper and black pepper.

Garlic Hummus

Serving size: ¼ cup
Servings per recipe: 8
Calories: ¼ cup
Preparation time: 10 minutes
Cooking time: 0 minutes

Ingredients:

- no-salt-added chickpeas (15 ounce)
- tahini ¼ cup
- extra-virgin olive oil ¼ cup
- lemon juice ¼ cup
- garlic clove 1
- ground cumin 1 teaspoon
- chili powder ½ teaspoon
- salt ½ teaspoon

Nutrition Information
Carbs: 9.7 g
Proteins: 3.7 g
Fats: 11.9 g

Instructions

1. Firstly drain chickpeas, reserve ¼ cup of the liquid. Shift the chickpeas and liquid reserved to a food processor. Now add lemon juice, tahini, oil, garlic, cumin, chilli powder and salt. Keep pureeing for 2-3 minutes or till very smooth.

Clementine & Pistachio Ricotta

Serving size: 2/3 cup
Servings per recipe: 1
Calories: 178
Preparation time: 2 minutes
Cooking time: 5 minutes

Ingredients:

- part-skim ricotta ⅓ cup

- peeled and segmented clementine, 1

- chopped pistachios 2 teaspoons

Nutrition Information

- ✓ **Carbs:** 14.6 g
- ✓ **Proteins:** 11.1 g
- ✓ **Fats:** 9 g

Instructions

1. Into a small bowl spoon ricotta and top it with clementine and pistachios.

Ricotta & Yogurt Parfait

Serving size: 1 ¼ cup
Servings per recipe: 1
Calories: 272
Preparation time: 2 minutes
Cooking time: 5 minutes

Ingredients:

- non-fat vanilla Greek yogurt ¾ cup

- part-skim ricotta ¼ cup

- lemon zest ½ teaspoon

- raspberries ¼ cup

- slivered almonds 1 tablespoon

- chia seeds 1 teaspoon

Nutrition Information
- ✓ **Carbs: 25.1 g**
- ✓ **Proteins: 21.7 g**
- ✓ **Fats: 9.6 g**

Instructions

1. In a bowl combine ricotta, yogurt and lemon zest. Do the topping with raspberries, almond and chia seeds.

Mediterranean Picnic Snacks

Serving size: 1 ¼ cup
Servings per recipe: 1
Calories: 197
Preparation time: 2 minutes
Cooking time: 3 minutes

Ingredients:

- Crusty whole-wheat bread slice-1, cut into bite size pieces
- Cherry tomatoes 10
- Sliced aged cheese ¼
  Oil cured olives 6

Nutrition Information
Carbs: 22 g
Proteins: 7.1 g
Fats: 9.1 g

Instructions

In a portable container combine bread pieces, cheese olives and tomatoes.

Crock Pot Chunky Monkey Paleo Trail Mix Recipe

Serving size: ¼ cup
Servings per recipe: 5-6 cups
Calories: 250
Preparation time: 5 minutes
Cooking time: 1 hour 30 minute

Ingredients:

- raw walnuts 2 cup (halves or coarsely chopped)
- raw cashews halves 1 cup (whole almonds work too)
- unsweetened coconut flakes 1 cup (be sure to get big FLAKES not shredded)
- coconut sugar 1/3 cup
- butter (cut in slices) 1– 1.5 tablespoon or at room temp 2 to 3 tablespoon coconut oil to make vegan
- vanilla or butter extract 1 tablespoon
- unsweetened banana chips or freeze dried banana slices 6 ounces
- dark chocolate chips or paleo fudge chunks 1/2 cup to 2/3 cup (we used Enjoy life foods brand)

Nutrition Information

Carbs: 18 g

Proteins: 4 g

Instructions

1. In a crockpot place nuts, coconut, sugar, vanilla, butter slices or coconut oil. Mix all these items and keep on high for 45-60 minutes. Don't forget to stir a few times, check in between to make sure coconut that coconut flakes do not burn. Lower the flame after 45 minutes if flakes cook faster or start turning brown.
2. Turn the flame to low and keep cooking for 20-30 minutes.
3. Take it off and place content of crock pot on parchment paper in order to dry out. Ensure that it is cooled for at the minimum 15 minutes prior to adding the chocolate and banana chips.
4. Now add in chocolate chips and banana chips and mix together.
5. Unsweetened banana chips can optionally be added to cook with coconut/nuts, instead of adding afterwards. But it will need stirring frequently. It must be cooked for 45 minutes only.
6. Store in a zip-lock bag or in an airtight container.

Savory Feta Spinach and Sweet Red Pepper Muffins

Serving size: 2
Servings per recipe: 12
Calories: 240 kcal
Preparation time: 10 minutes
Cooking time: 25 minutes

Ingredients:

- all purpose flour you can substitute partly with whole wheat flour 2 ¾
- cups sugar ¼ cup
- baking powder 2 teaspoons
- paprika 1 teaspoon
- salt ¾ teaspoon
- low fat milk ¾ cup
- extra virgin olive oil ½ cup
- eggs- 2
- fresh spinach 1 ¼ cup - thinly sliced
- crumbled feta ¾ cup
- Florina peppers or other red pepper 1/3 cup (drained and patted dry jarred)

Nutrition Information: Carbs: 13 g; Proteins: 4 g; Fats: 2 g

Instructions

1. Heat oven beforehand at 375 F.
2. Mix the dry ingredients: flour, sugar, baking powder, paprika and salt
3. Mix the olive oil, eggs and milk in another bowl.
4. Now add the wet ingredients to the dry ingredients and keep mixing until blended with a wooden spoon. The dough will become thick.
5. Mix gently after adding feta, spinach and peppers, continue till all ingredients are spread thoroughly in the whole mixture.
6. Now divide mixture in muffin pan that you have lined with cupcake/muffin liners. A silicon muffin tray and grease it with a little olive oil. But the oil should be enough for 12 medium muffins.
7. Next bake it for about 25 minutes. Take it off when toothpick comes out clear when inserted in the muffin.
8. Leave them to cool for 10 minutes and then take off from tray, let them cool a couple of hours before you serve it.

Smoked Salmon, Avocado and Cucumber Bites

Serving size: 3 bites
Servings per recipe: 12 bites
Calories: 46kcal
Preparation time: 2 minutes
Cooking time: 8 minutes

Ingredients:

- medium cucumber 1
- large avocado, peeled and pit removed 1
- lime juice 1/2 tablespoon
- smoked salmon 6 oz
- chives, for garnish
- black pepper, for garnish

Nutrition Information
Carbs: 2 g
Proteins: 2 g
Fats: 3 g

Instructions

1. Using a serrated knife slice the cucumber of about ¼ inch thick and lay flat on a service plate.

2. Next put the avocado and lime juice to a bowl and using a fork to mash until creamy.
3. Now assemble the bites and spread a small quantity of avocado on each cucumber, thereafter do topping with a thin slice of smoked salmon.
4. Now dress each bite with finely chopped chives and cracked black pepper. Serve at once.

Conclusion

Today what we desire the most is neither money nor palatial villas but the happiness by living a healthy life. Moreover, we are ready to pay any price for it and equally ready to follow any workout routine. However hard it may be. It is an established fact that there is a direct relationship in our fitness and the food we it. If this food is more plant-based and has good monosaturated fat along with protein. It is a blessing. If it is time tested, it is even better. This is what we find in Mediterranean diet. Going through all these recipes of diet routine—Breakfast, lunch, dinner and snacks, it becomes clear that there is no space for unhealthy fat, preservatives, refined sugar or flour. As all these food items tax different systems of our body. Further, it does not make a hole in your pocket and the ingredients too are easily available.

In the beginning it may be difficult to switch to Mediterranean diet completely. As it is said change is always difficult. But walking a step at a time can always make it possible. You can do it in the beginning by swapping any meal of the day—breakfast, lunch, dinner or even snacks. This diet will make you feel light and healthy—both physically and mentally. There is a science to it. The Mediterranean diet has little saturated fats or any other unhealthy fats. Its monosaturated fat boosts HDL, that is, the healthy cholesterol and keeps our coronary health strong. This is an input that keeps us on track while we follow this diet. As just by doing cardio alone you may not be able to keep your heart healthy by doing cardiovascular exercise alone. Reduced amount of weight would mean, less possibility of type 2 diabetes.

It is noticeable across all the recipes of the diet of people living in Mediterranean basin that it has either plants or fish. It means it has healthy meat and all natural ingredients that has protein, micro nutrients and fibre that makes our internal biological systems run smoothly. The fibre in it helps in cleaning our internal system and the antioxidants mints and vitamin c, B1, B2 and A rich items like quinoa, the chickpea which is rich in Vitamin D, has calcium etc. really ensures its health value. Similarly, there is a reign of fruits like banana, avocado, sweet potatoes; vegetables like tomato, spinach, broccoli, ginger, mushroom and garlic; dry fruits like pistachio, currants; when it comes to fats, there is only healthy fats that comes from olive oil. And the whole wheat and grains keeps you conscious of being full all through and handle those craving better.

The good news is there are lot many options and recipes that resemble items which decorate our platters today—pizza, muffins, salads, snacks, pitas, yogurt, dips etc. Moreover, one can choose easily among vegan, vegetarian and non-vegetarian. It shows following Mediterranean diet is easy and equally easy is to keep it implemented for long time. But we need to give it a start.

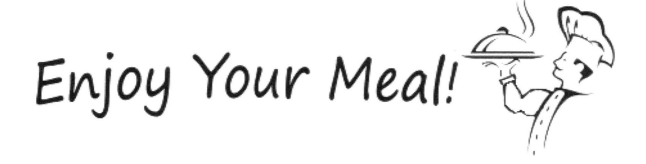

The Ultimate Keto Guide for Beginners after 50:

Cookbook with Tasty & Easy Recipes for a Healthy Life and Losing Weight Quickly. 21 Day Meal Plan to the Ketogenic Diet for Men and Women over 50.

|2021 Edition|

© Copyright 2021 by Weight Loss Academy

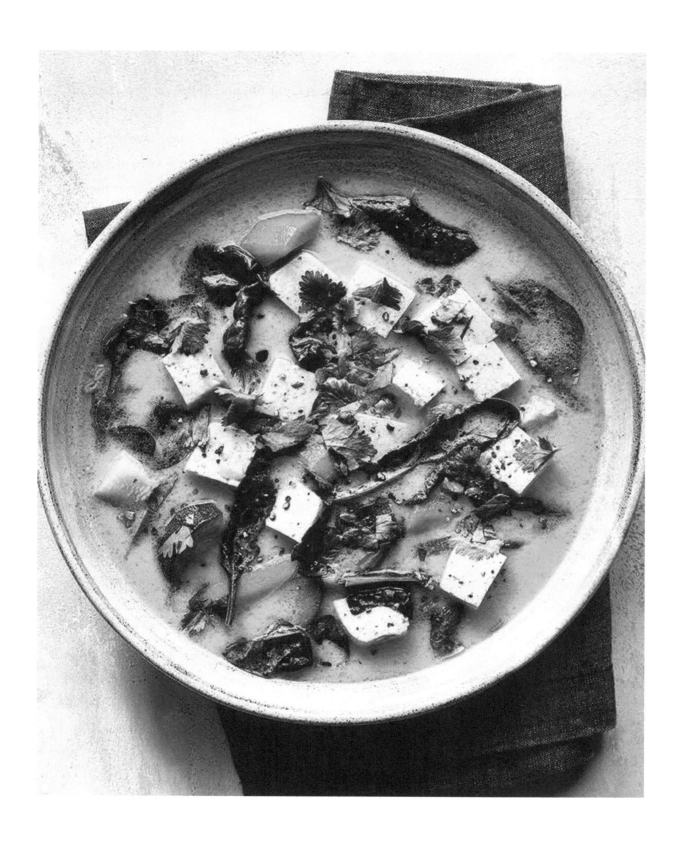

Introduction

Congratulations on purchasing **Keto Diet For Women Over 50**, and thank you for doing so.

This book is for women over 50 looking to lose weight and increase energy levels through the ketogenic (keto) diet. Naysayers will say the keto diet is a fad, but some form of this diet has been used for various health purposes, including weight loss, since 1825. Over the last 200 years, the diet has been changed and adjusted to incorporate the newest scientific information into the diet. As a result, the keto diet takes an age-old concept of limiting carbohydrates with the current knowledge of how fats work in the human body and now the diet is better than ever. The weight loss, when adapting the keto diet, is almost immediate. This book provides a basic framework for losing weight and improving your health by adopting a low-carbohydrate, high-fat diet. Your questions will be answered. By now, you've probably realized that it is not as easy to lose weight as it was when you were younger. That is probably the result of a lot of things; a slowing metabolism and decreased mobility are the obvious reasons you may be gaining weight, but the food you eat may be a culprit as well. Reading this book, you will be able to completely restructure your life and diet to follow ketogenic principles. The ketogenic diet is designed to help you lose weight with an increased energy level. This book outlines the basics and has the information to get you started. As a bonus, you will receive over 20 recipes that follow the keto diet principles. These recipes give you an opportunity to find new and creative ways to prepare food when you are starting out and may not be familiar with all the foods on the plan. There is also a food list inside that you can use to plan meals and purchase groceries for your new lighter, healthier lifestyle.

There happens to be a lot of books out there on this subject. Thank you for purchasing this one! I made sure it is jam packed with helpful information to get you where you want to be. Enjoy!

Is the Keto Diet Healthy for People Over 50?

The health benefits of the Keto diet are not different for men or women, but the speed at which they are reached does differ. As mentioned, human bodies are a lot different when it comes to the ways that they are able to burn fats and lose weight. For example, by design women have at least 10% more body fat than men. No matter how fit you are, this is just an aspect of being a human that you must consider. Don't be hard on yourself if you notice that it seems like men can lose weight easier that's because they can! What women have in additional body fat, men typically have the same in muscle mass. This is why men tend to see faster external results, because that added muscle mass means that their metabolism rates are higher. That increased metabolism means that fat and energy get burned faster. When you are on Keto, though, the internal change is happening right away.

Your metabolism is unique, but it is also going to be slower than a man's by nature. Since muscle is able to burn more calories than fat, the weight just seems to fall off of men, giving them the ability to reach the opportunity for muscle growth quickly. This should not be something that holds you back from starting your Keto journey. As long as you are keeping these realistic bodily factors in mind, you won't be left wondering why it is taking you a little bit longer to start losing weight. This point will come for you, but it will take a little bit more of a process that you must be committed to following through with.

Another unique condition that a woman can experience but a man cannot be PCOS or Polycystic Ovary Syndrome; a hormonal imbalance that causes the development of cysts. These cysts can cause pain, interfere with normal reproductive function, and, in extreme and dangerous cases, burst. PCOS is actually very common among women, affecting up to 10% of the entire female population. Surprisingly, most women are not even aware that they have the condition. Around 70% of women have PCOS that is undiagnosed. This condition can cause a significant hormonal imbalance, therefore affecting your metabolism. It can also inevitably lead to weight gain, making it even harder to see results while following diet plans. In order to stay on top of your health, you must make sure that you are going to the gynecologist regularly.

Menopause is another reality that must be faced by women, especially as we age. Most women begin the process of menopause in their mid-40s. Men do not go through menopause, so they are spared from yet another condition that causes slower metabolism and weight gain. When you start menopause, it is easy to gain weight and lose muscle. Most women, once menopause begins, lose muscle at a much faster rate, and conversely gain weight, despite dieting and exercise regimens. Keto can, therefore, be the right diet plan for you. Regardless of what your body is doing naturally, via processes like menopause, your internal systems are still going to be making the switch from running on carbs to deriving energy from fats.

When the body begins to run on fats successfully, you have an automatic fuel reserving waiting to be burned. It will take some time for your body to do this, but when it does, you will actually be able to eat fewer calories and still feel just as full because your body knows to take energy from the fat that you already have. This will become automatic. It is, however, a process that requires some patience, but being aware of what is actually going on with your body can help you stay motivated while on Keto.

Because a Keto diet reduces the amount of sugar you are consuming, it naturally lowers the amount of insulin in your bloodstream. This can actually have amazing effects on any existing PCOS and fertility issues, as well as menopausal symptoms and conditions like pre-diabetes and

Type 2 diabetes. Once your body adjusts to a Keto diet, you are overcoming the things that are naturally in place that can be preventing you from losing weight and getting healthy. Even if you placed your body on a strict diet, if it isn't getting rid of sugars properly, you likely aren't going to see the same results that you will when you try Keto. This is a big reason why Keto can be so beneficial for women.

You might not even realize that your hormones are not in balance until you experience a lifestyle that limits carbs and eliminates sugars. Keto is going to reset this balance for you, keeping your hormones at healthy levels. As a result of this, you will probably find yourself in a better general mood, and with much more energy to get through your days.

For people over 50, there are guidelines to follow when you start your Keto diet. As long as you are following the method properly and listening to what your body truly needs, you should have no more problems than men do while following the plan. What you will have are more obstacles to overcome, but you can do it. Remember that plenty of women successfully follow a Keto diet and see great results. Use these women as inspiration for how you anticipate your own journey to go. On the days when it seems impossible, remember what you have working against you, but more importantly what you have working for you. Your body is designed to go into ketogenesis more than it is designed to store fat by overeating carbs. Use this as a motivation to keep pushing you ahead. Keto is a valid option for you and the results will prove this, especially if you are over the age of 50.

The Keto Mistakes Everyone Makes

Do you feel like you are giving your all to the Keto diet but you still aren't seeing the results you want? You are measuring ketones, working out, and counting your macros, but you still aren't losing the weight you want. Here are the most common mistakes that most people make when beginning the Keto diet.

1. Too Many Snacks

There are many snacks you can enjoy while following the Keto diet, like nuts, avocado, seeds, and cheese. But, snacking can be an easy way to get too many calories into the diet while giving your body an easy fuel source besides stored fat. Snacks need to be only used if you frequently hunger between meals. If you aren't extremely hungry, let your body turn to your stored fat for its fuel between meals instead of dietary fat.

2. Not Consuming Enough Fat

The ketogenic diet isn't all about low carbs. It's also about high fats. You need to be getting about 75 percent of your calories from healthy fats, five percent from carbs, and 20 percent from protein. Fat makes you feel fuller longer, so if you eat the correct amount, you will minimize your carb cravings, and this will help you stay in ketosis. This will help your body burn fat faster.

3. Consuming Excessive Calories

You may hear people say you can eat what you want on the Keto diet as long as it is high in fat. Even though we want that to be true, it is very misleading. Healthy fats need to make up the biggest part of your diet. If you eat more calories than what you are burning, you will gain weight, no matter what you eat because these excess calories get stored as fat. An average adult only needs about 2,000 calories each day, but this will vary based on many factors like activity level, height, and gender.

4. Consuming a lot of Dairies

For many people, dairy can cause inflammation and keeps them from losing weight. Dairy is a combo food meaning it has carbs, protein, and fats. If you eat a lot of cheese as a snack for the fat content, you are also getting a dose of carbs and protein with that fat. Many people can olerate dairy, but moderation is the key. Stick with no more than one to two ounces of cheese or cream at each meal. Remember to factor in the protein content.

5. Consuming a lot of Protein

The biggest mistake that most people make when just beginning the Keto diet is consuming too much protein. Excess protein gets converted into glucose in the body called gluconeogenesis. This is a natural process where the body converts the energy from fats and proteins into glucose when glucose isn't available. When following a ketogenic diet, gluconeogenesis happens at different rates to keep body function. Our bodies don't need a lot of carbs, but we do need glucose. You can eat absolute zero carbs, and through gluconeogenesis, your body will convert other substances into glucose to be used as fuel. This is why carbs only make up five percent of your macros. Some parts of our bodies need carbs to survive, like kidney, medulla, and red blood cells. With gluconeogenesis, our bodies make and stores extra glucose as glycogen just in case supplies become too low.

In a normal diet, when carbs are always available, gluconeogenesis happens slowly because the need for glucose is extremely low. Our body runs on glucose and will store excess protein and carbs as fat.

6. Not Getting Enough Water

Water is crucial for your body. Water is needed for all your body does, and this includes burning fat. If you don't drink enough water, it can cause your metabolism to slow down, and this can halt your weight loss. Drinking 64 ounces or one-half gallon every day will help your body burn fat, flush out toxins, and circulate nutrients. When you are just beginning the Keto diet, you might need to drink more water since your body will begin to get rid of body fat by flushing it out through urine.

7. Consuming Too Many Sweets

Some people might indulge in Keto brownies and Keto cookies that are full of sugar substitute just because their net carb content is low, but you have to remember that you are still eating calories. Eating sweets might increase your carb cravings. Keto sweets are great on occasion; they don't need to be a staple in the diet.

8. Not Getting Enough Sleep

Getting plenty of sleep is needed in order to lose weight effectively. Without the right amount of sleep, your body will feel stressed, and this could result in your metabolism slowing down. It might cause it to store fat instead of burning fat. When you feel tired, you are more tempted to drink more lattes for energy, eat a snack to give you an extra boost, or order takeout rather than cooking a healthy meal. Try to get between seven and nine hours of sleep each night. Understand that your body uses that time to burn fat without you even lifting a finger.

9. Low on Electrolytes

Most people will experience the Keto flu when you begin this diet. This happens for two reasons when your body changes from burning carbs to burning fat, your brain might not have enough energy, and this, in turn, can cause grogginess, headaches, and nausea. You could be dehydrated, and your electrolytes might be low since the Keto diet causes you to urinate often.

Getting the Keto flu is a great sign that you are heading in the right direction. You can lessen these symptoms by drinking more water or taking supplements that will balance your electrolytes.

10. Consuming Hidden Carbs

Many foods look like they are low carb, but they aren't. You can find carbs in salad dressings, sauces, and condiments. Be sure to check nutrition labels before you try new foods to make sure it doesn't have any hidden sugar or carbs. It just takes a few seconds to skim the label, and it might be the difference between whether or not you'll lose weight.

If you have successfully ruled out all of the above, but you still aren't losing weight, you might need to talk with your doctor to make sure you don't have any health problems that could be preventing your weight loss. This can be frustrating, but stick with it, stay positive, and stay in

the game. When the Keto diet is done correctly, it is one of the best ways to lose weight.

How to Get into Ketosis

Ketogenic Vs Low Carb

Keto and low carbohydrate diets are similar in many ways. On a ketogenic diet, the body moves to a ketosis state, and the brain is ultimately powered by ketones. These are produced in the liver when the intake of carbohydrates is very small. Low carbohydrate diets may entail diverse things for different people. Low-carb diets actually reduce your overall carbohydrate consumption.

For regular low-carb diets, brain habits are still mostly glucose-dependent, although they may consume higher ketones than standard diets. To accomplish this, you'd have to follow low-carb, low-calorie, and an active lifestyle. The amount of carbohydrate you eat depends on the type of diet you consume.

At the end of the day, low carb is reduced in your carb intake. Mentions can vary enormously depending on the number of total carbs consumed per day. People have different views and follow different rules, from 0 to 100 grams of net carbs. Though a ketogenic diet has low carbohydrates, it also has significantly low protein levels. The overall increase in blood levels of ketones is significant.

What Is Ketosis?

When you reduce the intake of carbs over a period of time, the body can begin to break down body fat for energy for daily tasks. This is a natural occurrence called ketosis that the body undergoes to help us survive while food intake is small. We create ketones during this process, produced from the breakdown of fats in the liver. Once ketones are processed into energy, they are a byproduct of fatty acids.

Blood ketone bodies also increase substantially to higher than normal levels. Mind, muscle and all tissue that includes mitochondria utilize ketones. With practice, you'll soon learn how to understand ketosis signs.

A properly controlled ketogenic diet has the function of pushing your body into the metabolic state to consume fats as energy. Not by depriving the body of calories but by eliminating sugars. The bodies are outstandingly resilient to what you place in them. Taking keto nutrients such as keto OS can improve cell regeneration, strength, and lifespan. If an excess of fats is available, and carbs are eliminated, ketones can continue to burn as the primary source of energy.

Can A Keto Diet Help You Lose Weight?

There are different ways that a ketogenic diet will help a person shed excess fat in their body to meet their target weight. Scientists are still doing thorough research to understand just how this whole process works and how precisely the condition of ketosis helps an individual in terms of losing their excess weight.

Because protein intake is improved in most situations when a person moves to a ketogenic diet, and there are many healthy eating choices, including some veggies, that are filled with fiber in this specific type of diet, one of the most popular reasons would be better satiety. For fiber and protein, you'll find that you don't feel hungry as long as you've had a meal similar to before you had such same meals and you've decided to follow the diet.

With improved satiety and dieting plans, binge eating is something that can usually be avoided effectively. If you don't feel hungry between the main meals of the day, there's little need for a bag of potato chips or an energy bar.

Nonetheless, there would be moments where hunger hits—in such situations, carrying a handful of nuts can be a very healthy alternative to those energy bars, donuts, and other unhealthy, dangerous snacks that you normally choose when you find you need to consume when it's not time for the following meal.

Foods Allowed in Keto Diet

To make the most of your diet, there are prohibited foods, and others that are allowed, but in limited quantities. Here are the foods allowed in the ketogenic diet:

Food allowed in unlimited quantities
Lean or fatty meats
No matter which meat you choose, it contains no carbohydrates so that you can have fun! Pay attention to the quality of your meat, and the amount of fat. Alternate between fatty meats and lean meats!

Here are some examples of lean meats:

Beef: sirloin steak, roast beef, 5% minced steak, roast, flank steak, tenderloin, Grisons meat, tripe, kidneys

Horse: roti, steak

Pork: tenderloin, bacon, kidneys

Veal: cutlet, shank, tenderloin, sweetbread, liver

Chicken and turkey: cutlet, skinless thigh, ham

Rabbit

Here are some examples of fatty meats:

Lamb: leg, ribs, brain

Beef: minced steak 10, 15, 20%, ribs, rib steak, tongue, marrow

Pork: ribs, brain, dry ham, black pudding, white pudding, bacon, terrine, rillettes, salami, sausage, sausages, and merguez

Veal: roast, paupiette, marrow, brain, tongue, dumplings

Chicken and turkey: thigh with skin

Guinea fowl

Capon

Turkey

Goose: foie gras

Lean or fatty fish

The fish does not contain carbohydrates so that you can consume unlimited! As with meat, there are lean fish and fatty fish, pay attention to the amount of fat you eat and remember to vary your intake of fish. Oily fish have the advantage of containing a lot of good cholesterol, so it is beneficial for protection against cardiovascular disease! It will be advisable to consume fatty fish more than lean fish, to be able to manage your protein intake: if you consume lean fish, you will have a significant protein intake and little lipids, whereas with fatty fish, you will have a balanced protein and fat intake!

Here are some examples of lean fish:

1. Cod

2. Colin

3. Sea bream

4. Whiting

5. Sole

6. Turbot

7. Limor career

8. Location

9. Pike

10. Ray

Here are some examples of oily fish:

1. Swordfish

2. Salmon

3. Tuna

4. Trout

5. Monkfish

6. Herring

7. Mackerel

8. Cod

9. Sardine

Eggs

The eggs contain no carbohydrates, so you can consume as much as you want. It is often said that eggs are full of cholesterol and that you have to limit their intake, but the more cholesterol you eat, the less your body will produce by itself! In addition, it's not just poor-quality cholesterol so that you can consume 6 per week without risk! And if you want to eat more but you are afraid for your cholesterol and I have not convinced you, remove the yellow!

Vegetables and raw vegetables

Yes, you can eat vegetables. But you have to be careful which ones: you can eat leafy vegetables (salad, spinach, kale, red cabbage, Chinese cabbage...) and flower vegetables (cauliflower, broccoli, Romanesco cabbage...) as well as avocado, cucumbers, zucchini or leeks, which do not contain many carbohydrates.

The oils

It's oil, so it's only fat, so it's unlimited to eat, but choose your oil wisely! Prefer olive oil, rapeseed, nuts, sunflower or sesame for example!

Foods authorized in moderate quantities

The cold cuts
- As you know, there is bad cholesterol in cold meats, so you will need to moderate your intake:
- eat it occasionally!
- Fresh cheeses and plain yogurts
- Consume with moderation because they contain carbohydrates.
- Nuts and oilseeds

They have low levels of carbohydrates, but are rich in saturated fatty acids, that's why they should moderate their consumption. Choose almonds, hazelnuts, Brazil nuts or pecans.

Coconut (in oil, cream or milk)
It contains saturated fatty acids, that's why we limit its consumption. Cream and coconut oil contain a lot of medium chain triglycerides (MCTs), which increase the level of ketones, essential to stay in ketosis.

Berries and red fruits
They contain carbohydrates, in reasonable quantities, but you should not abuse them to avoid ketosis (blueberries, blackberries, raspberries...).

Benefit of Keto Diet for People Over 50

Benefits Ketogenic Diet

Reduction of cravings and appetite

Many people gain weight simply because they cannot control their cravings and appetite for caloric foods. The ketogenic diet helps eliminate these problems, but it does not mean that you will never be hungry or want to eat. You will feel hungry but only when you have to eat. Several studies have shown that the less carbohydrates you eat, the less you eat overall. Eating healthier foods that are high in fat helps reduce your appetite, as you lose more weight faster on a low-fat diet. The reason for this is that low carbohydrate diets help lower insulin levels, as your body does not need too much insulin to convert glycogen to glucose while eliminating excess water in your body. This diet helps you reduce visceral fat. In this way, you will get a slimmer look and shape. It is the most difficult fat to lose, as it surrounds the organs as it increases. High doses can cause inflammation and insulin resistance. Coconut oil can produce an immediate source of energy as it increases ketone levels in your body.

Reduction of risk of heart disease

Triglycerides, fat molecules in your body, have close links with heart disease. They are directly proportional as the more the number of triglycerides, the higher your chances of suffering from heart disease. You can reduce the number of free triglycerides in your body by reducing the number of carbohydrates, as is in the keto diets.

Reduces chances of having high blood pressure

Weight loss and blood pressure have a close connection; thus, since you are losing weight while on the keto diet, it will affect your blood pressure .

Fights type 2 diabetes

Type two diabetes develops as a result of insulin resistance. This is a result of having huge amounts of glucose in your system, with the keto diet this is not a possibility due to the low carbohydrate intake.

Increases the production of HDL

High-density lipoprotein is referred to as good cholesterol. It is responsible for caring calories to your liver, thus can be reused. High fat and low carbohydrate diets increase the production of HDL in your body, which also reduces your chances of getting a heart disease. Low-density lipoprotein is referred to as bad cholesterol.

Suppresses your appetite

It is a strange but true effect of the keto diet. It was thought that this was a result of the production of ketones but this was proven wrong as a study taken between people on a regular balanced diet and some on the keto diet and their appetites were generally the same. It, however, helps to suppress appetite as it is it has a higher fat content than many other diets. Food stays in the stomach for longer as fat and is digested slowly, thus provides a sense of fullness. On top of that, proteins promote the secretion cholecystokinin, which is a hormone that aids in regulating appetite. It is also believed that the ketogenic diet helps to suppress your appetite by continuous blunting of appetite. There is increased appetite in the initial stages of the diet, which decreases over time.

Changes in cholesterol levels

This is kind of on the fence between good and bad. This is because the ketogenic diet involves a high fat intake which makes people wonder about the effect on blood lipids and its potential to increase chances of heart disease and strokes, among others. Several major components play a lead role in determining this, which is: LDL, HDL, and blood triglyceride levels. Heart disease correlates with high levels of LDL and cholesterol.

On the other hand, high levels of HDL are seen as protection from diseases caused by cholesterol levels. The impacts of the diet on cholesterol are not properly known. Some research has shown that there is no change in cholesterol levels while others have said that there is change. If you stay in deep ketosis for a very long period of time, your blood lipids will increase, but you will have to go through some negative effects of the ketogenic diet which will be corrected when the diet is over. If a person does not remain following the diet strictly for like ten years, he/she will not experience any cholesterol problems. It is difficult to differentiate the difference between diet and weight loss in general.

The effect of the ketogenic diet on cholesterol has been boiled down to if you lose fat on the ketogenic diet then your cholesterol levels will go down, and if you don't lose fat, then your cholesterol levels will go up. Strangely, women have a larger cholesterol level addition than men, while both are on a diet. As there is no absolute conclusion on the effect of the ketogenic diet on cholesterol, you are advised to have your blood lipid levels constantly checked for any bad effects. Blood lipid levels should be checked before starting the diet and about eight weeks after starting. If repeated results show a worsening of lipid levels, then you should abandon the diet or substitute saturated fats with unsaturated fats.

Risk of a Ketogenic Diet

Low energy levels

When available, the body prefers to use carbohydrates for fuel as they burn more effectively than fats. General drop-in energy level is a concern raised by many dieters due to the lack of carbohydrates. Studies have shown that it causes orthostatic hypotension which causes lightheadedness. It has come to be known that these effects can be avoided by providing enough supplemental nutrients like sodium. Many of the symptoms can be prevented by providing 5 grams of sodium per day.

Most times, fatigue disappears after a few weeks or even days, if fatigue doesn't disappear, then you should add a small number of carbohydrates to the diet as long as ketosis is maintained. The diet is not recommended when caring out high-intensity workouts, weight training, or high-intensity aerobic exercise as carbohydrates are an absolute requirement but are okay for low-intensity exercise.

Effects on the brain

It causes increased use of ketones by the brain. The increased use of ketones, among other reasons, result in the treating of childhood epilepsy. As a result of the changes that occur, the concern over the side effects, including permanent brain damage and short-term memory loss, has been raised. The origin of these concerns is difficult to understand. The brain is powered by ketones in the absence of glucose. Ketones are normal energy sources and not toxic as the brain creates enzymes, during fetal growth, that helps us use them. Epileptic children, though not the perfect examples, show some insight into the effects of the diet on the brain in the long term. There is no negative effect in terms of cognitive function. There is no assurance that the diet cannot have long term dietary effects, but no information proves that there are any negative effects. Some people feel they can concentrate more when on the ketogenic diet, while others feel nothing but fatigue. This is as a result of differences in individual physiology. There are very few studies that vaguely address the point on short term memory loss. This wore off with the continuation of the study .

Kidney stones and kidney damage

As a result of the increased workload from having to filter ketones, urea, and ammonia, as well as dehydration concerns of the potential for kidney damage or passing kidney stones have been raised. The high protein nature of the ketogenic diet raises the alarms of individuals who are concerned with potential kidney damage. There is very little information that points to any negative effects of the diet on kidney function or development of kidney stones. There is a low incidence of small kidney stones in epileptic children this may be as a result of the state of deliberate dehydration that the children are put at instead of the ketosis state itself. Some short term research shows no change in kidney function or increased incidents of kidney stones either after they are off the diet or after six months on a diet.

There is no long term data on the effects of ketosis to kidney function; thus, no complete conclusions can be made. People with preexisting kidney issues are the only ones who get problems from high protein intake. From an unscientific point of view, one would expect increased incidents of this to happen to athletes who consume very high protein diets, but it has not happened. This suggests that high protein intake, under normal conditions, is not harmful to the kidneys. To limit the possibility of kidney stones, it is advised to drink a lot of water to maintain hydration. For people who are predisposed to kidney stones should have their kidney function should be monitored to ensure that no complications arise if they decide to follow through with the diet.

Constipation

A common side effect of the diet is reduced bowel movements and constipation. This arises from two different causes: lack of fiber and gastrointestinal absorption of foods. First, the lack of carbs in the diet means that unless supplements are taken, fiber intake is low. Fiber is very important to our systems. High fiber intake can prevent some health conditions, including heart disease and some forms of cancer. Use some type of sugar-free fiber supplement to prevent any health problems and help you maintain regular bowel movements. The diet also reduces the volume of stool due to enhanced absorption and digestion of food; thus, fewer waste products are generated.

Fat regain

Dieting, in general, has very low long term success rates. There are some effects of getting out of a ketogenic diet like the regain of fat lost through calorific restriction alone. This is true for any diet based on calorific restriction. It is expected for weight to be regained after carb reintroduction. For people who use the weighing scale to measure their success, they may completely shun carbs as they think it is the main reason for the weight regain. You should understand that most of the initial weight gain is water and glycogen.

Immune system

There is a large variety in the immunity system response to ketogenic diets on different people. There has been some repost on reduction on some ailments such allergies and increased minor sickness susceptibility.

Optic neuropathy

This is optic nerve dysfunction. It has appeared in a few cases, but it is still existence. It was linked to the people not getting adequate amounts of calcium or vitamins supplements for about a year. All the cases were corrected by supplementation of adequate vitamin B, especially thiamine.

Keto Grocery List

I've had people complain about the difficulty of switching their grocery list to one that's Ketogenic-friendly. The fact is that food is expensive – and most of the food you have in your fridge are probably packed full with carbohydrates. This is why if you're committing to a Ketogenic Diet, you need to do a clean sweep. That's right – everything that's packed with carbohydrates should be identified and set aside to make sure you're not eating more than you should. You can donate them to a charity before going out and buying your new Keto-friendly shopping list.

Seafood

Seafood means fish like sardines, mackerel, and wild salmon. It's also a good idea to add some shrimp, tuna, mussels, and crab into your diet. This is going to be a tad expensive but definitely worth it in the long run. What's the common denominator in all these food items? The secret is omega-3 fatty acids which is credited for lots of health benefits. You want to add food rich in omega-3 fatty acids in your diet.

Low-carb Vegetables

Not all vegetables are good for you when it comes to the Ketogenic Diet. The vegetable choices should be limited to those with low carbohydrate counts. Pack up your cart with items like spinach, eggplant, arugula, broccoli, and cauliflower. You can also put in bell peppers, cabbage, celery, kale, Brussels sprouts, mushrooms, zucchini, and fennel.

So what's in them? Well, aside from the fact that they're low-carb, these vegetable also contain loads of fiber which makes digestion easier. Of course, there's also the presence of vitamins, minerals, antioxidants, and various other nutrients that you need for day to day life. Which ones should you avoid? Steer clear of the starch-packed vegetables like carrots, turnips, and beets. As a rule, you go for the vegetables that are green and leafy.

Fruits Low in Sugar

During an episode of sugar-craving, it's usually a good idea to pick low-sugar fruit items. Believe it or not, there are lots of those in the market! Just make sure to stock up on any of these: avocado, blackberries, raspberries, strawberries, blueberries, lime, lemon, and coconut. Also note that tomatoes are fruits too so feel free to make side dishes or dips with loads of tomatoes! Keep in mind that these fruits should be eaten fresh and not out of a can. If you do eat them fresh off the can however, take a good look at the nutritional information at the back of the packaging. Avocadoes are particularly popular for those practicing the Ketogenic Diet because they contains LOTS of the good kind of fat.

Meat and Eggs

While some diets will tell you to skip the meat, the Ketogenic Diet actually encourages its consumption. Meat is packed with protein that will feed your muscles and give you a consistent source of energy through the day. It's a slow but sure burn when you eat protein as opposed to carbohydrates which are burned faster and therefore stored faster if you don't use them immediately.

But what kind of meat should you be eating? There's chicken, beef, pork, venison, turkey, and lamb. Keep in mind that quality plays a huge role here – you should be eating grass-fed organic beef or organic poultry if you want to make the most out of this food variety. The organic option lets you limit the possibility of ingesting toxins in your body due to the production process of these products. Plus, the preservation process also means there are added salt or sugar in the meat, which can throw off the whole diet.

Nuts and Seeds

Nuts and seeds you should definitely add in your cart include: chia seeds, Brazil nuts, macadamia nuts, flaxseed, walnuts, hemp seeds, pecans, sesame seeds, almonds, hazelnut, and pumpkin seeds. They also contain lots of protein and very little sugar so they're great if you have the munchies. They're the ideal snack because they're quick, easy, and will keep you full. They're high in calories though, which is why lots of people steer clear of them. As I mentioned earlier though – the Ketogenic Diet has nothing to do with calories and everything to do with the nutrient you're eating. So don't pay too much attention on the calorie count and just remember that they're a good source of fats and protein.

Dairy Products

OK – some people in their 50s already have a hard time processing dairy products, but for those who don't – you can happily add many of these to your diet. Make sure to consume sufficient amounts of cheese, plain Greek yogurt, cream butter, and cottage cheese. These dairy products are packed with calcium, protein, and the healthy kind of fat.

Oils

Nope, we're not talking about essentials oils but rather, MCT oil, coconut oil, avocado oil, nut oils, and even extra-virgin olive oil. You can start using those for your frying needs to create healthier food options. The beauty of these oils is that they add flavor to the food, making sure you don't get bored quickly with the recipes. Try picking up different types of Keto-friendly oils to add some variety to your cooking.

Coffee and Tea

The good news is that you don't have to skip coffee if you're going on a Ketogenic Diet. The bad news is that you can't go to Starbucks anymore and order their blended coffee choices. Instead, beverages would be limited to unsweetened tea or unsweetened coffee in order to keep the sugar consumption low. Opt for organic coffee and tea products to make the most out of these powerful antioxidants.

Dark Chocolate

Yes – chocolate is still on the menu, but it is limited to just dark chocolate. Technically, this means eating chocolate that is 70 percent cacao, which would make the taste a bit bitter.

Sugar Substitutes

Later in the recipes part of this book, you might be surprised at some of the ingredients required in the list. This is because while sweeteners are an important part of food preparation, you can't just use any kind of sugar in your recipe. Remember: the typical sugar is pure carbohydrate.

Even if you're not eating carbohydrates, if you're dumping lots of sugar in your food – you're not really following the Ketogenic Diet principles.

So what do you do? You find sugar substitutes. The good news is that there are LOTS of those in the market. You can get rid of the old sugar and use any of these as a good substitute.

Stevia. This is perhaps the most familiar one in this list. It's a natural sweetener derived from plants and contains very few calories. Unlike your typical sugar, stevia may actually help lower the sugar levels instead of causing it to spike. Note though that it's sweeter than actual sugar so when cooking with stevia, you'll need to lower the amount used. Typically, the ratio is 200 grams of sugar per 1 teaspoon of powdered stevia.

Sucralose. It contains zero calories and zero carbohydrates. It's actually an artificial sweetener and does not metabolize – hence the complete lack of carbohydrates. Splenda is actually a sweetener derived from sucralose. Note though that you don't want to use this as a baking substitute for sugar. Its best use is for coffee, yogurt, and oatmeal sweetening. Note though that like stevia, it's also very sweet – in fact, it's actually 600 times sweeter than the typical sugar. Use sparingly.

Erythritol. It's a naturally occurring compound that interacts with the tongue's sweet taste receptors. Hence, it mimics the taste of sugar without actually being sugar. It does contain calories, but only about 5% of the calories you'll find in the typical sugar. Note though that it doesn't dissolve very well so anything prepared with this sweetener will have a gritty feeling. This can be problematic if you're using the product for baking. As for sweetness, the typical ratio is 1 1/3 cup for 1 cup of sugar.

Xylitol. Like erythritol, xylitol is a type of sugar alcohol that's commonly used in sugar-free gum. While it still contains calories, the calories are just 3 per gram. It's a sweetener that's good for diabetic patients because it doesn't raise the sugar levels or insulin in the body. The great thing about this is that you don't have to do any computations when using it for baking, cooking, or fixing a drink. The ratio of it with sugar is 1 to 1 so you can quickly make the substitution in the recipe.

What about Condiments?

Condiments are still on the table, but they won't be as tasty as you're used to. Your options include mustard, olive oil mayonnaise, oil-based salad dressings, and unsweetened ketchup. Of all these condiments, ketchup is the one with the most sugar, so make a point of looking for one with reduced sugar content. Or maybe avoid ketchup altogether and stick to mustard?

What about Snacks?

The good news is that there are packed snacks for those who don't have the time to make it themselves. Sugarless nut butters, dried seaweeds, nuts, and sugar-free jerky are all available in stores. The nuts and seeds discussed in a previous paragraph all make for excellent snack options.

What about Labels?

Let's not fool ourselves into thinking that we can cook food every single day. The fact is that there will be days when there will be purchases for the sake of convenience. There are also instances when you'll have problems finding the right ingredients for a given recipe. Hence, you'll need to find substitutes for certain ingredients without losing the "Keto friendly" vibe of the product.

So what should be done? Well, you need to learn how to read labels. Food doesn't have to be specially made to be keto-friendly, you just have to make sure that it doesn't contain any of the unfriendly nutrients or that the carbohydrate content is low enough.

28 Days Meal Plan

Days	Breakfast	Lunch	Dinner	Snacks
1	Antipasti Skewers	Buttered Cod	Beef-Stuffed Mushrooms	Blueberry Scones
2	Kale, Edamame and Tofu Curry	Salmon with Red Curry Sauce	Rib Roast	Homemade Graham Crackers
3	Chocolate Cupcakes with Matcha Icing	Salmon Teriyaki	Beef Stir Fry	Buffalo Chicken Sausage Balls
4	Sesame Chicken Salad	Pesto Shrimp with Zucchini Noodles	Sweet & Sour Pork	Brussels Sprouts Chips
5	Jalapeno Poppers	Crab Cakes	Grilled Pork with Salsa	Keto Chocolate Mousse
6	BLT Party Bites	Tuna Salad	Garlic Pork Loin	Keto Berry Mousse
7	Strawberries and Cream Smoothie	Keto Frosty	Chicken Pesto	Peanut Butter Mousse
8	Cauli Flitters	Keto Shake	Garlic Parmesan Chicken Wings	Cookie Ice Cream
9	Bacon Wrapped Chicken Breast	Keto Fat Bombs	Crispy Baked Shrimp	Mocha Ice Cream
10	No-Bake Keto Power Bars	Avocado Ice Pops	Herbed Mediterranean Fish Fillet	Raspberry Cream Fat Bombs
11	Avocado Toast	Carrot Balls	Mushroom Stuffed with Ricotta	Cauliflower Tartar Bread
12	Almond Flour Pancakes	Coconut Crack Bars	Thai Chopped Salad	Buttery Skillet Flatbread
13	Chicken Avocado Egg Bacon Salad	Buttered Cod	Lemon & Rosemary Salmon	Fluffy Bites
14	Keto Flu Combat Smoothie	Strawberry Ice Cream	Chicken Kurma	Coconut Fudge

15	Bacon Hash	Key Lime Pudding	Pork Chops with Bacon & Mushrooms	Nutmeg Nougat
16	Egg Salad	Chicken, Bacon and Avocado Cloud Sandwiches	Pork	Sweet Almond Bites
17	Bagels with Cheese	Roasted Lemon Chicken Sandwich	Garlic Shrimp	Strawberry Cheesecake Minis
18	Capicola Egg Cups	Keto-Friendly Skillet Pepperoni Pizza	Pork Chop	Cocoa Brownies
19	Scrambled Eggs	Cheesy Chicken Cauliflower	Citrus Egg Salad	Blueberry Scones
20	Frittata with Spinach	Chicken Soup	Chowder	Homemade Graham Crackers
21	Cheese Omelet	Chicken Avocado Salad	Beef-Stuffed Mushrooms	Buffalo Chicken Sausage Balls
22	Antipasti Skewers	Chicken Broccoli Dinner	Rib Roast	Brussels Sprouts Chips
23	Kale, Edamame and Tofu Curry	Easy Meatballs	Beef Stir Fry	Keto Chocolate Mousse
24	Chocolate Cupcakes with Matcha Icing	Chicken Casserole	Sweet & Sour Pork	Keto Berry Mousse
25	Sesame Chicken Salad	Lemon Baked Salmon	Grilled Pork with Salsa	Peanut Butter Mousse
26	Jalapeno Poppers	Italian Sausage Stacks	Garlic Pork Loin	Cookie Ice Cream
27	BLT Party Bites	Baked Salmon	Chicken Pesto	Mocha Ice Cream
28	Strawberries and Cream Smoothie	Tuna Patties	Garlic Parmesan Chicken Wings	Raspberry Cream Fat Bombs

Breakfast

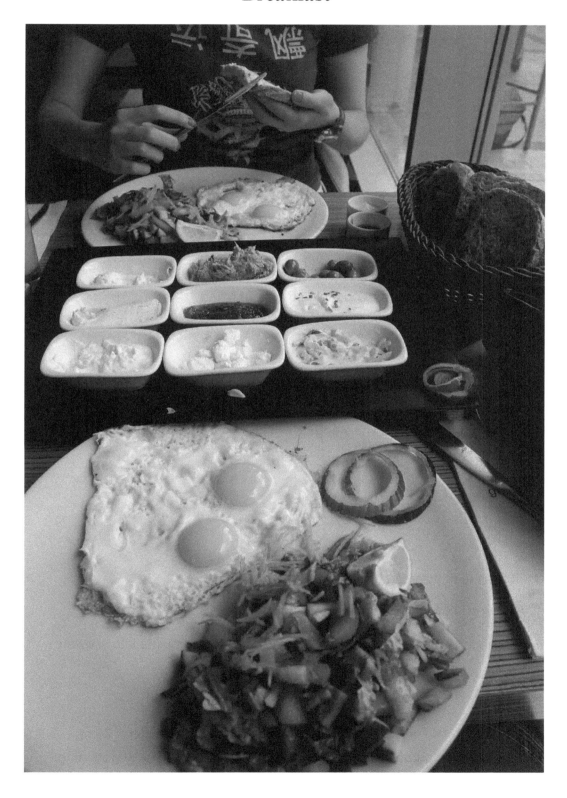

Antipasti Skewers

Preparation Time: 10 minutes
Cooking Time: 0 minute
Servings: 6

Ingredients:

- 6 small mozzarella balls

- 1 tablespoon olive oil

- Salt to taste

- 1/8 teaspoon dried oregano

- 2 roasted yellow peppers, sliced into strips and rolled

- 6 cherry tomatoes

- 6 green olives, pitted

- 6 Kalamata olives, pitted

- 2 artichoke hearts, sliced into wedges

- 6 slices salami, rolled

- 6 leaves fresh basil

Directions:

1. Toss the mozzarella balls in olive oil.

2. Season with salt and oregano.

3. Thread the mozzarella balls and the rest of the ingredients into skewers.

4. Serve in a platter.

Nutrition: Calories 180; Total Fat 11.8g; Saturated Fat 4.5g; Cholesterol 26mg ; Sodium 482mg; Total Carbohydrate 11.7g; Dietary Fiber 4.8g; Total Sugars 4.1g; Protein 9.2g; Potassium 538mg

Kale, Edamame and Tofu Curry

Preparation Time: 20 minutes
Cooking Time: 40 minutes
Servings: 3

Ingredients:

- tablespoon rapeseed oil
- 1 large onion, chopped
- Four cloves garlic, peeled and grated
- 1 large thumb (7cm) fresh ginger, peeled and grated
- 1 red chili, deseeded and thinly sliced
- 1/2 teaspoon ground turmeric
- 1/4 teaspoon cayenne pepper
- 1 teaspoon paprika
- 1/2 teaspoon ground cumin

- 1 teaspoon salt
- 250 g / 9 oz. dried red lentils
- 1-liter boiling water
- 50 g / 1.7 oz. frozen soya beans
- 200 g / 7 oz. firm tofu, chopped into cubes
- Two tomatoes, roughly chopped
- Juice of 1 lime
- 200 g / 7 oz. kale leaves stalk removed and torn

Directions:

1. Put the oil in a pan over low heat. Add your onion and cook for 5 minutes before adding the garlic, ginger, and chili and cooking for a further 2 minutes. Add your turmeric, cayenne, paprika, cumin, and salt and Stir through before adding the red lentils and stirring again.
2. Pour in the boiling water and allow it to simmer for 10 minutes, reduce the heat and cook for about 20-30 minutes until the curry has a thick '•porridge' consistency.
3. Add your tomatoes, tofu and soya beans and cook for a further 5 minutes. Add your kale leaves and lime juice and cook until the kale is just tender.

Nutrition:

- ✓ Calories 133
- ✓ Carbohydrate 54
- ✓ Protein 43

Chocolate Cupcakes with Matcha Icing

Preparation Time: 35 minutes
Cooking Time: 0 minutes
Servings: 4

Ingredients:

- 150g / 5 oz. self-rising flour
- 200 g / 7 oz. caster sugar
- 60 g / 2.1 oz. cocoa
- ½ teaspoon. salt
- ½ teaspoon. fine espresso coffee, decaf if preferred 120 ml / ½ cup milk
- ½ teaspoon. vanilla extract
- 50 ml / ¼ cup vegetable oil
- egg
- 120 ml / ½ cup of water
- For the icing:
- 50 g / 1.7 oz. butter,
- 50 g / 1.7 oz. icing sugar
- 1 tablespoon matcha green tea powder
- ½ teaspoon vanilla bean paste
- 50 g / 1.7 oz. soft cream cheese

Directions:

1. Heat the oven and Line a cupcake tin with paper
2. Put the flour, sugar, cocoa, salt, and coffee powder in a large bowl and mix well.
3. Add milk, vanilla extract, vegetable oil, and egg to dry ingredients and use an electric mixer to beat until well combined. Gently pour the boiling water slowly and beat on low speed until completely combined. Use the high speed to beat for another minute to add air to the dough. The dough is much more liquid than a normal cake mix. Have faith; It will taste fantastic!
4. Arrange the dough evenly between the cake boxes. Each cake box must not be more than ¾ full. Bake for 15-18 minutes, until the dough resumes when hit. Remove from oven and allow cooling completely before icing.
5. To make the icing, beat your butter and icing sugar until they turn pale and smooth. Add the matcha powder and vanilla and mix again. Add the cream cheese and beat until it is smooth. Pipe or spread on the cakes.

Nutrition: calories435; Fat 5; Fiber 3; Carbs 7; Protein 9

Sesame Chicken Salad

Preparation Time: 20 minutes
Cooking Time: 0 minutes
Servings: 4

Ingredients

- tablespoon of sesame seeds
- 1 cucumber, peeled, halved lengthwise, without a teaspoon, and sliced.
- 100 g / 3.5 oz. cabbage, chopped
- 60 g pak choi, finely chopped
- ½ red onion, thinly sliced
- Large parsley (20 g / 0.7 oz.), chopped.
- 150 g / 5 oz. cooked chicken, minced
- For the dressing:
- 1 tablespoon of extra virgin olive oil
- 1 teaspoon of sesame oil
- 1 lime juice
- 1 teaspoon of light honey
- teaspoons soy sauce

Directions:

1. Roast your sesame seeds in a dry pan for 2 minutes until they become slightly golden and fragrant.
2. Transfer to a plate to cool.
3. In a small bowl, mix olive oil, sesame oil, lime juice, honey, and soy sauce to prepare the dressing.
4. Place the cucumber, black cabbage, pak choi, red onion, and parsley in a large bowl and mix gently.
5. Pour over the dressing and mix again.
6. Distribute the salad between two dishes and complete with the shredded chicken. Sprinkle with sesame seeds just before serving.

Nutrition:

- Calories 345
- Fat 5
- Fiber 2
- Carbs 10
- Protein 4

Jalapeno Poppers

Preparation Time: *30 minutes*
Cooking Time: *60 minutes*
Servings: *10*

Ingredients:

- 5 fresh jalapenos, sliced and seeded
- 4 oz. package cream cheese
- ¼ lb. bacon, sliced in half

Directions:

6. Preheat your oven to 275 degrees F.
7. Place a wire rack over your baking sheet.
8. Stuff each jalapeno with cream cheese and wrap in bacon.
9. Secure with a toothpick.
10. Place on the baking sheet.
11. Bake for 1 hour and 15 minutes.

Nutrition:

Calories 103

Total Fat 8.7g

Saturated Fat 4.1g

Cholesterol 25mg

Sodium 296mg

Total Carbohydrate 0.9g

Dietary Fiber 0.2g

Total Sugars 0.3g

Protein 5.2g

Potassium 93mg

BLT Party Bites

Preparation Time: *35 minutes*
Cooking Time: *0 minute*
Servings: *8*

Ingredients:

- 4 oz. bacon, chopped
- 3 tablespoons panko breadcrumbs
- tablespoon Parmesan cheese, grated
- 1 teaspoon mayonnaise
- 1 teaspoon lemon juice
- Salt to taste
- ½ heart Romaine lettuce, shredded
- 6 cocktail tomatoes

Directions:

5. Put the bacon in a pan over medium heat.
6. Fry until crispy.
7. Transfer bacon to a plate lined with paper towel.
8. Add breadcrumbs and cook until crunchy.
9. Transfer breadcrumbs to another plate also lined with paper towel.
10. Sprinkle Parmesan cheese on top of the breadcrumbs.
11. Mix the mayonnaise, salt and lemon juice.
12. Toss the Romaine in the mayo mixture.
13. Slice each tomato on the bottom to create a flat surface so it can stand by itself.
    Slice the top off as well.
    Scoop out the insides of the tomatoes.

Stuff each tomato with the bacon, Parmesan, breadcrumbs and top with the lettuce.

Nutrition:

Calories 107; Total Fat 6.5g; Saturated Fat 2.1g; Cholesterol 16mg; Sodium 360mg
Total Carbohydrate 5.4g ; Dietary Fiber 1.5g; Total Sugars 3.3g; Protein 6.5g
Potassium 372mg

Strawberries and Cream Smoothie

Preparation Time: *5 minutes*
Cooking Time: 15 minutes
Servings: 1

Ingredients:

- 5 medium strawberries, hulled
- 3 tablespoons heavy (whipping) cream
- 3 ice cubes
- Your favorite vanilla-flavored sweetener

Directions:

1. In a blender, combine all the ingredients and blend until smooth. Enjoy right away!

Nutrition:
Calories: 176
Total Fat: 16g
Protein: 2g
Total Carbs: 6g
Fiber: 1g
Net Carbs: 5g

Cauli Flitters

Preparation Time: 10 minutes

Cooking Time: 15 minutes

Servings: 2

Ingredients:

- 2 eggs
- 1 head of cauliflower
- 1 tbsp. yeast
- sea salt, black pepper
- 1-2 tbsp. ghee
- 1 tbsp. turmeric
- 2/3 cup almond flour

Directions:

10. Place the cauliflower into a large pot and start to boil it for 8 mins. Add the florets into a food processor and pulse them.
11. Add the eggs, almond flour, yeast, turmeric, salt and pepper to a mixing bowl. Stir well. Form into patties.
12. Heat your ghee to medium in a skillet. Form your fritters and cook until golden on each side (3-4 mins).
13. Serve it while hot.

Nutrition:

Calories: 238 kcal

Fat: 23 g

Carbs: 5 g

Protein: 6 g

Bacon Wrapped Chicken

Preparation Time: 10 minutes

Cooking Time: 45 minutes

Servings: 4

Ingredients

- 4 boneless, skinless chicken breast
- 8 oz. sharp cheddar cheese
- 8 slices bacon
- 4 oz. sliced jalapeno peppers
- 1 tsp garlic powder
- Salt and pepper to taste

Directions

7. Preheat the oven at around 3500F. Ensure to season both sides of chicken breast well with salt, garlic powder, and pepper. Place the chicken breast on a non-stick baking sheet (foil-covered). Cover the chicken with cheese and add jalapeno slices. Cut the bacon slices in half and then place the four halves over each piece of chicken. Bake for around 30 to 45 minutes at most. If the chicken is set but the bacon still feels undercooked, you may want to put it under the broiler for a few minutes. Once done, serve hot with a side of low carb garlic parmesan roasted asparagus.

Nutrition:

Calories: 640

Fat: 48g

Carbohydrates: 6g

Fiber: 3g

Net carbs: 3g

Protein: 47g

No-Bake Keto Power Bars

Preparation Time: 10 Minutes plus Overnight to Chill

Cooking Time: 20 minutes

Servings: 12 bars

Ingredients:

- ½ cup pili nuts
- ½ cup whole hazelnuts
- ½ cup walnut halves
- ¼ cup hulled sunflower seeds
- ¼ cup unsweetened coconut flakes or chips
- ¼ cup hulled hemp seeds
- 2 tablespoons unsweetened cacao nibs
- 2 scoops collagen powder (I use 1 scoop Perfect Keto vanilla collagen and
- 1 scoop Perfect Keto unflavored collagen powder)
- ½ teaspoon ground cinnamon
- ½ teaspoon sea salt
- ¼ cup coconut oil, melted
- teaspoon vanilla extract
- Stevia or monk fruit to sweeten (optional if you are using unflavored collagen powder)

Directions:

1. Line a 9-inch square baking pan with parchment paper.
2. In a food processor or blender, combine the pili nuts, hazelnuts, walnuts, sunflower seeds, coconut, hemp seeds, cacao nibs, collagen powder, cinnamon, and salt and pulse a few times.
3. Add the coconut oil, vanilla extract, and sweetener (if using). Pulse again until the ingredients are combined. Do not over pulse or it will turn to mush. You want the nuts and seeds to have some texture still.
4. Pour the mixture into the prepared pan and press it into an even layer. Cover with another piece of parchment (or fold over extra from the first piece) and place a heavy pan or dish on top to help press the bars together.
5. Refrigerate overnight and then cut into 12 bars. Store the bars in individual storage bags in the refrigerator for a quick grab-and-go breakfast.

Nutrition: Calories: 242; Total Fat: 22g; Protein: 6.5g; Total Carbs: 4.5g; Fiber: 2.5g

Net Carbs: 2g

Lunch

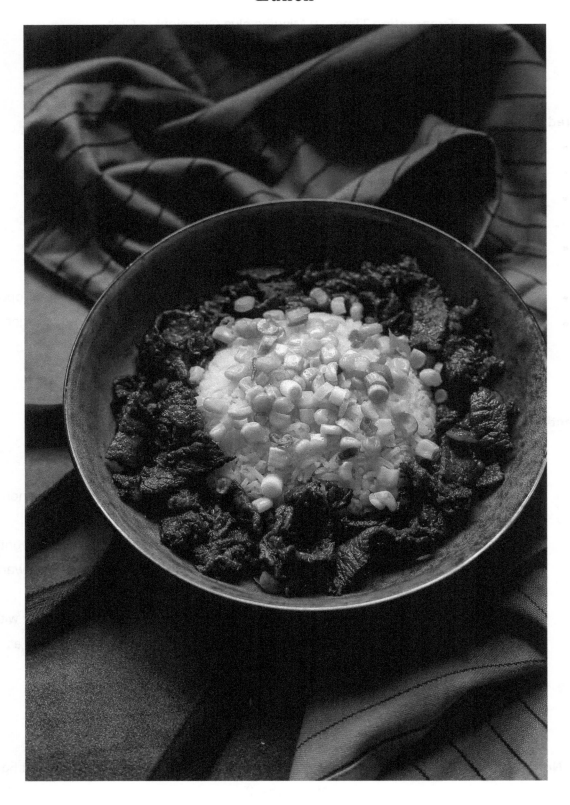

Buttered Cod

Preparation Time: *5 minutes*
Cooking Time: *5 minutes*
Servings: *4*

Ingredients:

1 ½ lb. cod fillets, sliced

6 tablespoons butter, sliced

¼ teaspoon garlic powder

¾ teaspoon ground paprika

Salt and pepper to taste

Lemon slices

Chopped parsley

Directions:

6. Mix the garlic powder, paprika, salt and pepper in a bowl.
7. Season cod pieces with seasoning mixture.
8. Add 2 tablespoons butter in a pan over medium heat.
9. Let half of the butter melt.
10. Add the cod and cook for 2 minutes per side.
11. Top with the remaining slices of butter.
12. Cook for 3 to 4 minutes.
13. Garnish with parsley and lemon slices before serving.

Nutrition:

1. Calories 295
2. Total Fat 19g
3. Saturated Fat 11g
4. Cholesterol 128mg
5. Sodium 236mg
6. Total Carbohydrate 1.5g
7. Dietary Fiber 0.7g
8. Total Sugars 0.3g
9. Protein 30.7g
10. Potassium 102mg

Salmon with Red Curry Sauce

Preparation Time: *10 minutes*
Cooking Time: *22 minutes*
Servings: *4*

Ingredients:

- 4 salmon fillets
- 2 tablespoons olive oil
- Salt and pepper to taste
- 1 ½ tablespoons red curry paste
- 1 tablespoon fresh ginger, chopped
- 14 oz. coconut cream
- 1 ½ tablespoons fish sauce

Directions:

3. Preheat your oven to 350 degrees F.
4. Cover baking sheet with foil.
5. Brush both sides of salmon fillets with olive oil and season with salt and pepper.
6. Place the salmon fillets on the baking sheet.
7. Bake salmon in the oven for 20 minutes.
8. In a pan over medium heat, mix the curry paste, ginger, coconut cream and fish sauce.
9. Sprinkle with salt and pepper.
10. Simmer for 2 minutes.
11. Pour the sauce over the salmon before serving.

Nutrition:

- ✓ Calories 553
- ✓ Total Fat 43.4g
- ✓ Saturated Fat 24.1g
- ✓ Cholesterol 78mg
- ✓ Sodium 908mg
- ✓ Total Carbohydrate 7.9g
- ✓ Dietary Fiber 2.4g
- ✓ Total Sugars 3.6g
- ✓ Protein 37.3g
- ✓ Potassium 982mg

Salmon Teriyaki

Preparation Time: *15 minutes*
Cooking Time: *25 minutes*
Servings: *6*

Ingredients:

- 3 tablespoons sesame oil
- 2 teaspoons fish sauce
- 3 tablespoons coconut amino
- 2 teaspoons ginger, grated
- 4 cloves garlic, crushed
- 2 tablespoons xylitol
- 1 tablespoon green lime juice
- 2 teaspoons green lime zest
- Cayenne pepper to taste
- 6 salmon fillets
- 1 teaspoon arrowroot starch
- ¼ cup water
- Sesame seeds

Directions:

6. Preheat your oven to 400 degrees F.
7. Combine the sesame oil, fish sauce, coconut amino, ginger, garlic, xylitol, green lime juice, zest and cayenne pepper in a mixing bowl.
8. Create 6 packets using foil.
9. Add half of the marinade in the packets.
10. Add the salmon inside.
11. Place in the baking sheet and cook for about 20 to 25 minutes.
12. Add the remaining sauce in a pan over medium heat.
13. Dissolve arrowroot in water, and add to the sauce.
14. Simmer until the sauce has thickened.
    Place the salmon on a serving platter and pour the sauce on top.
    Sprinkle sesame seeds on top before serving.

Pesto Shrimp with Zucchini Noodles

Preparation Time: 10 minutes

Cooking Time: 15 minutes

Servings: 3

Ingredients:

- Pesto sauce
- 3 cups basil leaves
- ¾ cup pine nuts
- 2 cloves garlic
- ½ lemon, juiced
- 1 teaspoon lemon zest
- Salt to taste
- ¼ cup olive oil
- Shrimp and Zoodles
- 3 zucchinis
- Salt to taste
- 1 lb. shrimp
- 2 tablespoons avocado oil

Directions:

4. Put all the pesto ingredients in a blender.
5. Blend until smooth.
6. Spiralize the zucchini into noodle form.
7. Season with salt.
8. Drain water from the zucchini noodles.
9. Season the shrimp with salt and pepper.
10. Add half of the oil in a pan over medium heat.
11. Once the oil is hot, add the shrimp and cook for 1 to 2 minutes.
12. Add the remaining oil to the pan.

    Add the zucchini noodles and cook for 3 minutes.

    Add the pesto and toss to coat the noodles evenly with the sauce.

    Season with salt.

Crab Cakes

Preparation Time: *1 hour and 20 minutes*
Cooking Time: *20 minutes*
Servings: *8*

Ingredients:

- 2 tablespoons butter

- 2 cloves garlic, minced

- ½ cup bell pepper, chopped

- 1 rib celery, chopped

- 1 shallot, chopped

- Salt and pepper to taste

- 2 tablespoons mayonnaise

- 1 egg, beaten

- 1 teaspoon mustard

- 1 tablespoon Worcestershire sauce

- 1 teaspoon hot sauce

- ½ cup Parmesan cheese, grated

- ½ cup pork rinds, crushed

- 1 lb. crabmeat

- 2 tablespoons olive oil

Directions:

1. Add the butter to the pan over medium heat.

2. Add the garlic, bell pepper, celery, shallot, salt and pepper.

3. Cook for 10 minutes.

4. In a bowl, mix the mayo, egg, Worcestershire, mustard and hot sauce.

5. Add the sautéed vegetables to this mixture.

6. Mix well.

7. Add the cheese and pork rind.

8. Fold in the crabmeat.

9. Line the baking sheet with foil.

10. Create patties from the mixture.

11. Place the patties on the baking sheet.

12. Cover the baking sheet with foil.

13. Refrigerate for 1 hour.

14. Fry in olive oil in a pan over medium heat.

15. Cook until crispy and golden brown.

Nutrition:
Calories 150
Total Fat 9.2g
Saturated Fat 3.2g
Cholesterol 43mg
Sodium 601mg
Total Carbohydrate 10.8g
Dietary Fiber 0.5g
Total Sugars 4.6g
Protein 6.4g
Potassium 80mg

Tuna Salad

Preparation Time: *5 minutes*
Cooking Time: *0 minute*
Servings: *2*

Ingredients:

- 1 cup tuna flakes
- 3 tablespoons mayonnaise
- 1 teaspoon onion flakes
- Salt and pepper to taste
- 3 cups Romaine lettuce

Directions:

8. Mix the tuna flakes, mayonnaise, onion flakes, salt and pepper in a bowl.
9. Serve with lettuce.

Nutrition:

Calories 130

Total Fat 7.8g

Saturated Fat 1.1g

Cholesterol 13mg

Sodium 206mg

Total Carbohydrate 8.5g

Dietary Fiber 0.6g

Total Sugars 2.6g

Protein 8.2g

Potassium 132mg

Keto Frosty

Preparation Time: 45 minutes

Cooking Time: 0 minute

Servings: 4

Ingredients:

- 1 ½ cups heavy whipping cream
- 2 tablespoons cocoa powder (unsweetened)
- 3 tablespoons Swerve
- 1 teaspoon pure vanilla extract
- Salt to taste

Directions:

9. In a bowl, combine all the ingredients.
10. Use a hand mixer and beat until you see stiff peaks forming.
11. Place the mixture in a Ziploc bag.
12. Freeze for 35 minutes.
13. Serve in bowls or dishes.

Nutrition:

Calories 164

Total Fat 17g

Saturated Fat 10.6g

Cholesterol 62mg

Sodium 56mg

Total Carbohydrate 2.9g

Dietary Fiber 0.8g

Total Sugars 0.2g

Protein 1.4g

Potassium 103mg

Keto Shake

Ingredients:

- ¾ cup almond milk
- ½ cup ice
- 2 tablespoons almond butter
- 2 tablespoons cocoa powder (unsweetened)
- 2 tablespoons Swerve
- 1 tablespoon chia seeds
- 2 tablespoons hemp seeds
- ½ tablespoon vanilla extract
- Salt to taste

Directions:

5. Blend all the ingredients in a food processor.
6. Chill in the refrigerator before serving.

Nutrition:

Calories 104

Potassium 159mg

Total Fat 9.5g

Saturated Fat 5.1g

Cholesterol 0mg

Sodium 24mg

Total Carbohydrate 3.6g

Dietary Fiber 1.4g

Total Sugars 1.1g

Protein 2.9g

Keto Fat Bombs

Preparation Time: *30 minutes*
Cooking Time: *0 minute*
Servings: *10*

Ingredients:

- 8 tablespoons butter
- ¼ cup Swerve
- ½ teaspoon vanilla extract
- Salt to taste
- 2 cups almond flour
- 2/3 cup chocolate chips

Directions:

9. In a bowl, beat the butter until fluffy.
10. Stir in the sugar, salt and vanilla.
11. Mix well.
12. Add the almond flour.
13. Fold in the chocolate chips.
14. Cover the bowl with cling wrap and refrigerate for 20 minutes.
15. Create balls from the dough.

Nutrition:

Calories 176

Total Fat 15.2g

Saturated Fat 8.4g

Cholesterol 27mg

Sodium 92mg

Total Carbohydrate 12.9g

Dietary Fiber 1g

Total Sugars 10.8g

Protein 2.2g

Potassium 45mg

Avocado Ice Pops

Preparation Time: *20 minutes*
Cooking Time: *0 minute*
Servings: *10*

Ingredients:

- 3 avocados
- ¼ cup lime juice
- 3 tablespoons Swerve
- ¾ cup coconut milk
- 1 tablespoon coconut oil
- 1 cup keto friendly chocolate

Directions:

4. Add all the ingredients except the oil and chocolate in a blender.
5. Blend until smooth.
6. Pour the mixture into the popsicle mold.
7. Freeze overnight.
8. In a bowl, mix oil and chocolate chips.
9. Melt in the microwave. And then let cool.
10. Dunk the avocado popsicles into the chocolate before serving.

Nutrition:

Calories 176

Total Fat 17.4g

Saturated Fat 7.5g

Cholesterol 0mg

Sodium 6mg

Total Carbohydrate 10.8g

Dietary Fiber 4.5g

Total Sugars 5.4g

Protein 1.6g

Potassium 341mg

Dinner

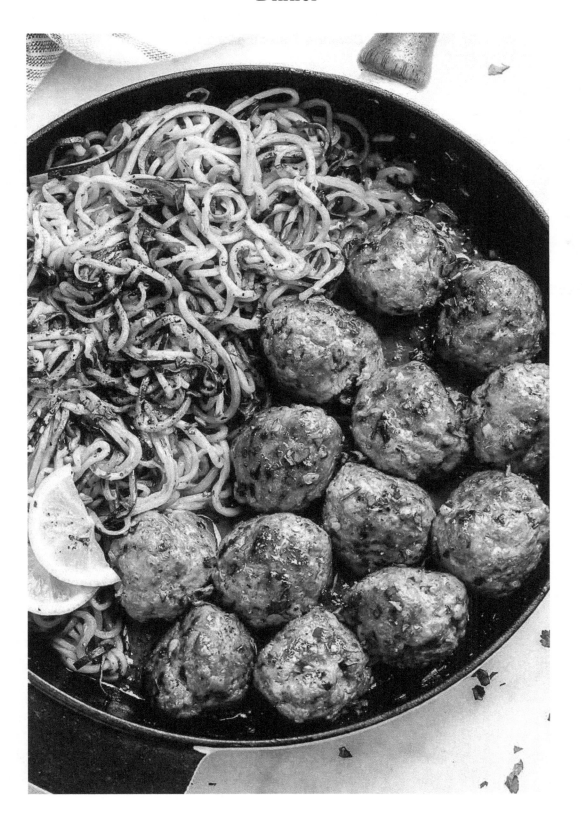

Beef-Stuffed Mushrooms

Preparation Time: 20 minutes

Cooking Time: 25 minutes

Servings: 4

Ingredients:

- 4 mushrooms, stemmed
- 3 tablespoons olive oil, divided
- 1 yellow onion, sliced thinly
- 1 red bell pepper, sliced into strips
- 1 green bell pepper, sliced into strips
- Salt and pepper to taste
- 8 oz. beef, sliced thinly
- 3 oz. provolone cheese, sliced
- Chopped parsley

Directions:

2   Preheat your oven to 350 degrees F.

3   Arrange the mushrooms on a baking pan.

4   Brush with oil.

5   Add the remaining oil to a pan over medium heat.

6   Cook onion and bell peppers for 5 minutes.

7   Season with salt and pepper.

8   Place onion mixture on a plate.

9   Cook the beef in the pan for 5 minutes.

10 Sprinkle with salt and pepper.

2.   Add the onion mixture back to the pan.

3.   Mix well.

4.   Fill the mushrooms with the beef mixture and cheese.

5.   Bake in the oven for 15 minutes.

Nutrition: Calories 333; Total Fat 20.3 g; Saturated Fat 6.7 g; Cholesterol 61 mg; Sodium 378 mg; Total Carbohydrate 8.2 g; Dietary Fiber 3.7 g; Protein 25.2 g; Total Sugars 7 g; Potassium 789 mg

Rib Roast

Preparation Time: 15 minutes

Cooking Time: 3 hours

Servings: 8

Ingredients:

- 1 rib roast
- Salt to taste
- 12 cloves garlic, chopped
- 2 teaspoons lemon zest
- 6 tablespoons fresh rosemary, chopped
- 5 sprigs thyme

Directions:

6. Preheat your oven to 325 degrees F.
7. Season all sides of rib roast with salt.
8. Place the rib roast in a baking pan.
9. Sprinkle with garlic, lemon zest and rosemary.
10. Add herb sprigs on top.
11. Roast for 3 hours.

Let rest for a few minutes and then slice and serve.

Nutrition:

1. Calories 329
2. Total Fat 27 g
3. Saturated Fat 9 g
4. Cholesterol 59 mg
5. Sodium 498 mg
6. Total Carbohydrate 5.3 g
7. Dietary Fiber 1.8 g
8. Protein 18 g
9. Total Sugars 2 g
10. Potassium 493 mg

Beef Stir Fry

Preparation Time: *15 minutes*

Cooking Time: *10 minutes*

Servings: *4*

Ingredients:

- 1 tablespoon soy sauce
- 1 tablespoon ginger, minced
- 1 teaspoon cornstarch
- 1 teaspoon dry sherry
- 12 oz. beef, sliced into strips
- 1 teaspoon toasted sesame oil
- 2 tablespoons oyster sauce
- 1 lb. baby bok choy, sliced
- 3 tablespoons chicken broth

Directions:

4. Mix soy sauce, ginger, cornstarch and dry sherry in a bowl.
5. Toss the beef in the mixture.
6. Pour oil into a pan over medium heat.
7. Cook the beef for 5 minutes, stirring.
8. Add oyster sauce, bok choy and chicken broth to the pan.
9. Cook for 1 minute.

Nutrition:

Calories 247

Total Fat 15.8 g

Saturated Fat 4 g

Cholesterol 69 mg

Sodium 569 mg

Total Carbohydrate 6.3 g

Dietary Fiber 1.1 g

Protein 25 g

Sweet & Sour Pork

Preparation Time: *15 minutes*

Cooking Time: *15 minutes*

Servings: *4*

Ingredients:

- 1 lb. pork chops
- Salt and pepper to taste
- ½ cup sesame seeds
- 2 tablespoons peanut oil
- 2 tablespoons soy sauce
- 3 tablespoons apricot jam
- Chopped scallions

Directions:

2 Season pork chops with salt and pepper.

3 Press sesame seeds on both sides of pork.

4 Pour oil into a pan over medium heat.

5 Cook pork for 3 to 5 minutes per side.

6 Transfer to a plate.

7 In a bowl, mix soy sauce and apricot jam.

8 Simmer for 3 minutes.

9 Pour sauce over the pork and garnish with scallions before serving.

Nutrition:

Calories 414

Total Fat 27.5 g

Saturated Fat 5.6 g

Cholesterol 68 mg

Sodium 607 mg

Total Carbohydrate 12.9 g

Dietary Fiber 1.8 g

Protein 29 g

Total Sugars 9 g

Potassium 332 mg

Grilled Pork with Salsa

Preparation Time: *30 minutes*

Cooking Time: *15 minutes*

Servings: *4*

Ingredients:

- Salsa
- 1 onion, chopped
- 1 tomato, chopped
- 1 peach, chopped
- 1 apricot, chopped
- 1 tablespoon olive oil
- 1 tablespoon lime juice
- 2 tablespoons fresh cilantro, chopped
- Salt and pepper to taste
- Pork
- 1 lb. pork tenderloin, sliced
- 1 tablespoon olive oil
- Salt and pepper to taste
- ½ teaspoon ground cumin
- ¾ teaspoon chili powder

Directions:

4. Combine salsa ingredients in a bowl.
5. Cover and refrigerate.
6. Brush pork tenderloin with oil.
7. Season with salt, pepper, cumin and chili powder.

8. Grill pork for 5 to 7 minutes per side.
9. Slice pork and serve with salsa.

Nutrition:

Calories 219; Total Fat 9.5 g; Saturated Fat 1.8 g; Cholesterol 74 mg;

Sodium 512 mg; Total Carbohydrate 8.3 g; Dietary Fiber 1.5 g; Protein 24 g; Total Sugars 6 g

Potassium 600 mg

Garlic Pork Loin

Preparation Time: *15 minutes*
Cooking Time: *1 hour*
Servings: *6*

Ingredients:

- 1 ½ lb. pork loin roast
- 4 cloves garlic, sliced into slivers
- Salt and pepper to taste

Directions:

7. Preheat your oven to 425 degrees F.
8. Make several slits all over the pork roast.
9. Insert garlic slivers.
10. Sprinkle with salt and pepper.
11. Roast in the oven for 1 hour.

Nutrition:

Calories 235

Total Fat 13.3 g

Saturated Fat 2.6 g

Cholesterol 71 mg

Sodium 450 mg

Total Carbohydrate 1.7 g

Dietary Fiber 0.3 g

Protein 25.7 g

Total Sugars 3 g

Potassium 383 mg

Chicken Pesto

Preparation Time: *15 minutes*
Cooking Time: *25 minutes*
Servings: *4*

Ingredients:

- 1 lb. chicken cutlet
- Salt and pepper to taste
- 1 tablespoon olive oil
- ½ cup onion, chopped
- ½ cup heavy cream
- ½ cup dry white wine
- 1 tomato, chopped
- ¼ cup pesto
- 2 tablespoons basil, chopped

Directions:

1. Season chicken with salt and pepper.
2. Pour oil into a pan over medium heat.
3. Cook chicken for 3 to 4 minutes per side.
4. Place the chicken on a plate.
5. Add the onion to the pan.
6. Cook for 1 minute.
7. Stir in the rest of the ingredients.
8. Bring to a boil.
9. Simmer for 15 minutes.
10. Put the chicken back to the pan.
11. Cook for 2 more minutes and then serve.

Nutrition:

Calories 371; Total Fat 23.7 g; Saturated Fat 9.2 g; Cholesterol 117 mg;
Sodium 361 mg; Total Carbohydrate 5.7 g; Dietary Fiber 1 g; Protein 27.7 g;
Total Sugars 3 g; Potassium 567 mg

Garlic Parmesan Chicken Wings

Preparation Time: 20 minutes
Cooking Time: 20 minutes
Servings: 8

Ingredients:

- Cooking spray
- ½ cup all-purpose flour
- Pepper to taste
- 2 tablespoons garlic powder
- 3 eggs, beaten
- ¼ cups Parmesan cheese, grated
- cups breadcrumbs
- lb. chicken wings

Directions:

1. Preheat your oven to 450 degrees F.
2. Spray baking pan with oil.
3. In a bowl, mix the flour, pepper and garlic powder.
4. Add eggs to another bowl.
5. Mix the Parmesan cheese and breadcrumbs in another bowl.
6. Dip the chicken wings in the first, second and third bowls.
7. Spray chicken wings with oil.
8. Bake in the oven for 20 minutes.

Nutrition:

1. Calories 221
2. Total Fat 11.6 g
3. Saturated Fat 3.9 g
4. Cholesterol 122 mg
5. Sodium 242 mg

6. Total Carbohydrate 8 g
7. Dietary Fiber 0.4 g

8. Protein 16 g
9. Total Sugars 3 g
10. Potassium 163 mg

Crispy Baked Shrimp

Preparation Time: *15 minutes*

Cooking Time: *10 minutes*

Servings: *4*

Ingredients:

- ¼ cup whole-wheat breadcrumbs
- 3 tablespoons olive oil, divided
- ½ lb. jumbo shrimp, peeled and deveined
- Salt and pepper to taste
- tablespoons lemon juice
- 1 tablespoon garlic, chopped
- tablespoons butter
- ¼ cup Parmesan cheese, grated
- 2 tablespoons chives, chopped

Directions:

6. Preheat your oven to 425 degrees F.
7. Add breadcrumbs to a pan over medium heat.
8. Cook until toasted.
9. Transfer to a plate.
10. Coat baking pan with 1 tablespoon oil.
11. Arrange shrimp in a single layer in a baking pan.
12. Season with salt and pepper.
13. Mix lemon juice, garlic and butter in a bowl.
14. Pour mixture on top of the shrimp.

    Add Parmesan cheese and chives to the breadcrumbs.

    Sprinkle breadcrumbs on top of the shrimp.

    Bake for 10 minutes.

Nutrition:

Calories 340; Total Fat 18.7 g; Saturated Fat 6 g; Cholesterol 293 mg;

Sodium 374 mg; Total Carbohydrate 6 g; Dietary Fiber 0.8 g; Protein 36.9 g

Total Sugars 2 g; Potassium 483 mg

Herbed Mediterranean Fish Fillet

Preparation Time: 20 minutes

Cooking Time: 1 hour

Servings: 6

Ingredients:

- 3 lb. sea bass fillet
- Salt to taste
- 2 tablespoons tarragon, chopped
- ¼ cup dry white wine
- 3 tablespoons olive oil, divided
- tablespoon butter
- cloves garlic, minced
- cups whole-wheat breadcrumbs
- tablespoons parsley, chopped
- 3 tablespoons oregano, chopped
- 3 tablespoons fresh basil, chopped

Directions:

2. Preheat your oven to 350 degrees F.
3. Season fish with salt and tarragon.
4. Pour half of oil into a roasting pan.
5. Stir in wine.
6. Add the fish in the roasting pan.
7. Bake in the oven for 50 minutes.
8. Add remaining oil to a pan over medium heat.
9. Cook herbs, breadcrumbs and salt.
10. Spread breadcrumb mixture on top of fish and bake for 5 minutes.

Nutrition:

Calories 288; Total Fat 12.7 g; Saturated Fat 2.9 g; Cholesterol 65 mg;

Sodium 499 mg Total Carbohydrate 10.4 g; Dietary Fiber 1.8 g; Protein 29.5 g

Total Sugars 1 g; Potassium 401 mg

Vegetables

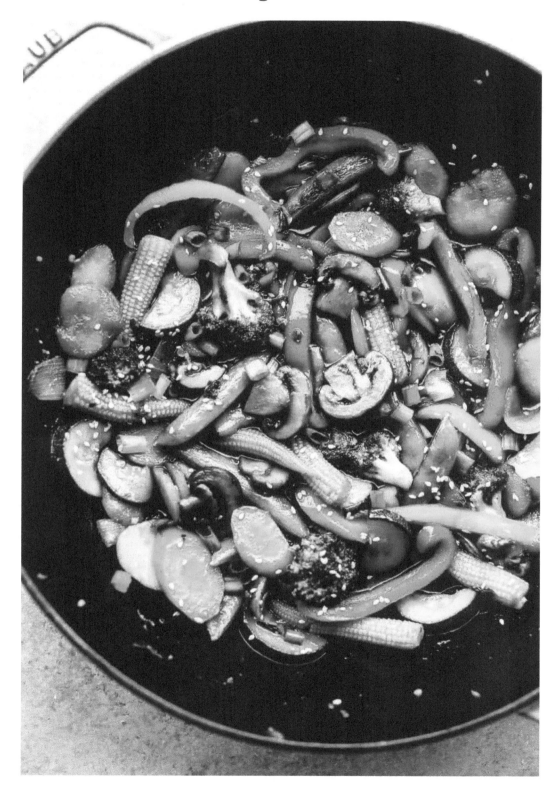

Tomato and broccoli soup

Preparation Time: 50 minutes

Cooking Time: 55 minutes

Servings: 4

Ingredients:

- A drizzle of olive oil
- Canned sugar-free tomatoes- 28 oz.
- Crushed red pepper- ¼ tsp.
- Broccoli head: into florets- 1
- Small ginger: chopped- 1
- Onion: chopped – 1
- Garlic clove: minced- 1
- Coriander seeds- 2 tsp.
- Black pepper
- Salt

Directions:

1. Boil water and salt in a pan on medium-high and add broccoli florets to steam for 2 minutes.
2. Remove and put in a bowl of ice water. Drain and set aside.
3. Heat pan and put in coriander seeds to toast for 4 minutes. Blend in a blender and set aside.
4. Pour olive oil in a pot and set to medium and add red pepper, salt, pepper and onions and cook for 7 minutes.
5. Mix in coriander seeds and garlic and let it cook for 3 minutes.
6. Pour in tomatoes and let simmer for 10 minutes.
7. Mix in broccoli and cook for 12 minutes.
8. Serve

Nutrition:

Calories- 152, carbs- 1, protein- 9, fiber- 8, fats- 9

Bok Choy Stir Fry with Fried Bacon Slices

Preparation Time: 17 minutes
Cooking Time: 15 minutes
Servings: 2

Ingredients:

- Bok choy; chopped - 2 cup.
- Garlic cloves; minced - 2Bacon slices; chopped - 2
- A drizzle of avocado oil
- Salt and black pepper to the taste.

Instructions:

1. Take a pan and heat it with oil over medium heat.
2. When the oil is hot, add bacon and keep stirring it until it's brown and crispy.
3. Transfer them to paper towels to drain out the excess oil.
4. Now bring the pan to medium heat and in it add garlic and bok choy.
5. Again give it a stir and cook it for 5 minutes.
6. Now drizzle and add some salt, pepper and the fried bacon and stir them for another 1 minute.
7. Turn off the heat and divide them in plates to serve.

Nutrition
Calories: 50; Fat: 1; Fiber: 1; Carbs: 2; Protein: 2

Broccoli-cauliflower stew

Preparation Time: 25 minutes
Cooking Time: 15 minutes
Servings: 5

Ingredients:

- Bacon slices: chopped -2
- Cauliflower head: separated into florets- 1
- Broccoli head: separated into florets- 1
- Butter- 2 tbsp.
- Garlic cloves: minced- 2
- Salt
- Black pepper

Directions:

1. Put a pan on medium heat and dissolve the butter and the garlic. Add the bacon slices to brown for 3 minutes all over.
2. Mix in broccoli and cauliflower florets to cook for 2 minutes.
3. Pour water over it and cover the lid and let cook for 10 minutes.
4. Season with pepper and salt and puree soup with a dipping blend.
5. Let boil slowly for some minutes on medium heat.
6. Serve into bowls.

Nutrition:

Calories- 128, carbs- 4, protein- 6, fiber- 7, fats- 2

Creamy Avocado Soup

Preparation Time: 20 minutes

Cooking Time: 15 minutes

Servings: 4

Ingredients:

- Chicken stock, 3 c.
- Black pepper
- Chopped scallions, 2
- Salt
- Heavy cream, 2/3 c.
- Butter, 2 tbsps.
- Chopped avocados, 2

Directions:

1. Over a medium source of heat, set the saucepan and cook the scallions for 2 minutes

2. Stir in 2 ½ cups stock to simmer for 3 minutes
3. Set the blender in position to blend avocados, heavy cream, the remaining stock, and seasonings.
4. Return to a pan to cook for 2 minutes as you adjust the seasoning
5. Serve in soup bowls

Nutrition:

Calories: 335, Fat: 32, Fiber: 9, Carbs: 13, Protein: 3

Bok choy mushroom soup

Preparation Time: 25 minutes

Cooking Time: 15 minutes

Servings: 4

Ingredients:

- Bacon strips: chopped- 2
- Beef stock- 3 cups
- Bok choy: chopped- 1 bunch
- Onion: chopped- 1
- Parmesan cheese: grated- 3 tbsp.
- Coconut aminos- 3 tbsp.
- Worcestershire sauce- 2 tbsp.
- Red pepper flakes- ½ tbsp.
- Mushrooms: chopped- 1½ cups
- Black Pepper
- Salt

Directions:

1. Put bacon in a saucepan over medium-high heat to brown until crispy then remove to paper towels to drain.
2. To medium heat, add the mushrooms and onions in the pan and cook for 15 minutes.
3. Pour in the stock, pepper flakes, aminos, bok choy, Worcestershire sauce, salt and pepper and mix.
4. Cook until bok choy is tender.
5. Serve into bowls and sprinkle with Parmesan cheese and bacon.

Nutrition:

Calories- 100, carbs- 1, protein- 5, fiber- 9, fats- 5

Tasty Radish Soup

Preparation Time: 30 minutes
Cooking Time: 45 minutes
Servings: 4

Ingredients:

- Chopped onion, 1
- Salt
- Chopped celery stalk, 2
- Chicken stock, 6 c.
- Coconut oil, 3 tbsps.
- Quartered radishes, 2 bunches
- Black pepper
- Minced garlic cloves, 6

Directions:

1. Set the pan over medium heat and melt the oil
2. Stir in the celery, onion, and garlic to cook until soft, about 5 minutes
3. Stir in the stock, radishes, and seasonings.
4. Cover and simmer to boil for 15 minutes
5. Enjoy while still hot

Nutrition:

Calories: 131, Fat: 12, Fiber: 8, Carbs: 4, Protein: 1

Fried garlicy bacon and bok choy broth

Preparation Time: 17 minutes
Cooking Time: 15 minutes
Servings: 2

Ingredients:

- Bok choy: chopped- 2 cups
- A drizzle of avocado oil
- Bacon slices: chopped- 2
- Garlic cloves: minced- 2
- Black pepper
- Salt

Directions:

1. Put bacon in a pan on medium heat and let crisp. Remove and let drain on paper towels.
2. Add bok choy and garlic to the pan and let cook for 4 minutes.
3. Season with pepper and salt and put the bacon back into the pan.
4. Let cook for 1 minute and serve.

Nutrition:

Calories- 116, carbs- 8, protein- 3, fiber- 8, fats- 1

Nutritional Mustard Greens and Spinach Soup

Preparation Time: 25 minutes

Cooking Time: 15 minutes

Servings: 6

Ingredients:

- Spinach; torn - 5 cups.
- Fenugreek seeds - 1/2 teaspoon.
- Cumin seeds - 1 teaspoon.
- Jalapeno; chopped - 1 tablespoon.
- Mustard greens; chopped - 5 cups.
- Ghee - 2 teaspoons.
- Paprika - 1/2 teaspoon.
- Avocado oil - 1 tablespoon.
- Coriander seeds - 1 teaspoon.
- Yellow onion; chopped - 1 cup.
- Garlic; minced - 1 tablespoon.
- Ginger; grated - 1 tablespoon.
- Turmeric; ground - 1/2 teaspoon.
- Coconut milk - 3 cups.
- Salt and black pepper to the taste.

Directions:

1. Add coriander, fenugreek and cumin seed in a heated pot with oil over medium high heat.
2. Now stir and brow them for 2 minutes.
3. In the same pot, add onions and again stir them for 3 minutes.
4. Now after the onion's cooked, add half of the garlic, jalapenos, ginger and turmeric.
5. Again, give it a good stir and cook for another 3 minutes.
6. Add some more mustard greens, spinach and saute everything for 10 minutes.
7. After it's done add milk, salt, pepper before blending the soup with an immersion blender.
8. Now take another pan and heat it up over medium heat with some ghee drizzled on it.
9. In it, add garlic, paprika, and give it a good stir before turning off the heat.
10. Bring the soup to heat over medium heat and transfer them into soup bowls.
11. Top it with some drizzles of ghee and paprika. Now it's ready to serve hot.

Hash Browns with Radish

Preparation Time: 20 minutes

Cooking Time: 15 minutes

Servings: 4

Ingredients:

- Shredded Parmesan cheese, 1/3 c.
- Garlic powder, ½ tsp.
- Salt
- Shredded radishes, 1 lb.
- Black pepper
- Onion powder, ½ tsp.
- Medium eggs, 4

Directions:

1. Set a large mixing bowl in a working surface.
2. Combine the seasonings, radishes, eggs, onion, and parmesan cheese
3. Arrange the mixture in a well-lined baking tray.
4. Set the oven for 10 minutes at 3750F. Allow to bake
5. Enjoy while still hot

Nutrition:

Calories: 104, Fat: 6, Fiber: 8, Carbs: 5, Protein: 6

Baked Radishes

Preparation Time: 30 minutes
Cooking Time: 35 minutes
Servings: 4

Ingredients:

- Chopped chives, 1 tbsp.
- Sliced radishes, 15
- Salt
- Vegetable oil cooking spray
- Black pepper

Directions:

1. Line your baking sheet well then spray with the cooking spray
2. Set the sliced radishes on the baking tray then sprinkle with cooking oil
3. Add the seasonings then top with chives
4. Set the oven for 10 minutes at 375oF, allow to bake
5. Turn the radishes to bake for 10 minutes
6. Serve cold

Nutrition:

Calories: 63, Fat: 8, Fiber: 3, Carbs: 6, Protein: 1

Poultry

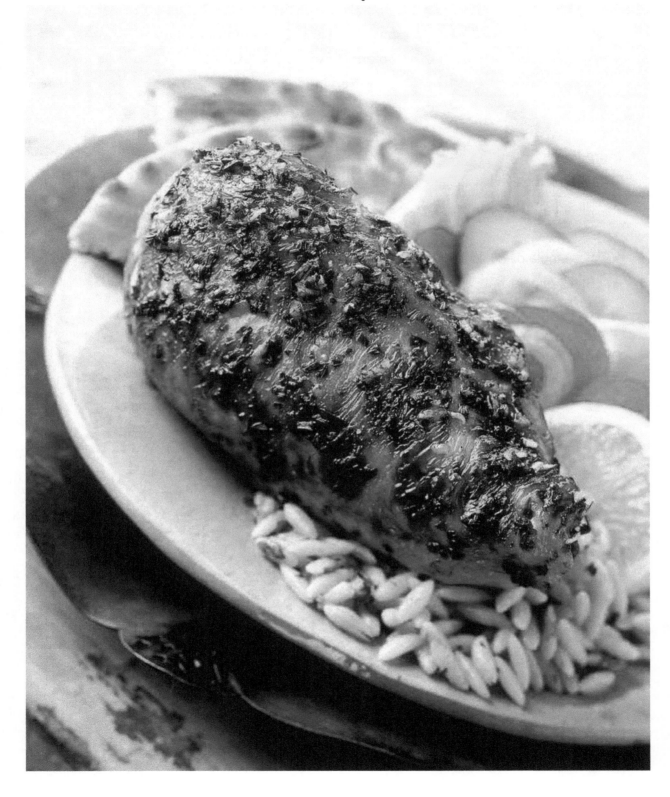

Pancakes

Preparation Time: 5 minutes
Cooking Time: 6 minutes
Servings: 2

Ingredients

- ¼ cup almond flour
- ½ tbsp. unsalted butter
- oz. cream cheese, softened
- eggs

Directions:

1. Take a bowl, crack eggs in it, whisk well until fluffy, and then whisk in flour and cream cheese until well combined.
2. Take a skillet pan, place it over medium heat, add butter and when it melts, drop pancake batter in four sections, spread it evenly, and cook for 2 minutes per side until brown.
3. Serve.

Nutrition :

166.8 Calories; 15 g Fats; 5.8 g Protein; 1.8 g Net Carb; 0.8 g Fiber;

Cheese Roll-Ups

Preparation Time: 5 minutes

Cooking Time: 0 minutes;

Servings: 2

Ingredients

- 2 oz. mozzarella cheese, sliced, full-fat
- 1-ounce butter, unsalted

Directions:

1.   Cut cheese into slices and then cut butter into thin slices.

2.   Top each cheese slice with a slice of butter, roll it and then serve .

Nutrition : 166 Calories; 15 g Fats; 6.5 g Protein; 2 g Net Carb; 0 g Fiber;

Scrambled Eggs with Spinach and Cheese

Preparation Time: 5 minutes

Cooking Time: 5 minutes;

Servings: 2

Ingredients

- 2 oz. spinach
- 2 eggs
- tbsp. coconut oil
- tbsp. grated mozzarella cheese, full-fat
- Seasoning:
- ¼ tsp salt
- 1/8 tsp ground black pepper
- 1/8 tsp red pepper flakes

Directions:

1. Take a medium bowl, crack eggs in it, add salt and black pepper and whisk until combined.
2. Take a medium skillet pan, place it over medium heat, add oil, add spinach and cook for 1 minute until leaves wilt.
3. Pour eggs over spinach, stir and cook for 1 minute until just set.
4. Stir in cheese, then remove the pan from heat and sprinkle red pepper flakes on top.

5. Serve.

Nutrition : 171 Calories; 14 g Fats; 9.2 g Protein; 1.1 g Net Carb; 1.7 g Fiber;

Egg Wraps

Preparation Time: 5 minutes
Cooking Time: 5 minutes;
Servings: 2

Ingredients

- 2 eggs
- tbsp. coconut oil
- Seasoning:
- ¼ tsp salt
- 1/8 tsp ground black pepper

Directions:

1. Take a medium bowl, crack eggs in it, add salt and black pepper, and then whisk until blended.
2. Take a frying pan, place it over medium-low heat, add coconut oil and when it melts, pour in half of the egg, spread it evenly into a thin layer by rotating the pan and cook for 2 minutes.
3. Then flip the pan, cook for 1 minute, and transfer to a plate.
4. Repeat with the remaining egg to make another wrap, then roll each egg wrap and serve.

Nutrition : 68 Calories; 4.7 g Fats; 5.5 g Protein; 0.5 g Net Carb; 0 g Fiber;

Chaffles with Poached Eggs

Preparation Time: 5 minutes

Cooking Time: 10 minutes;

Servings: 2

Ingredients

- 2 tsp coconut flour
- ½ cup shredded cheddar cheese, full-fat
- 3 eggs
- Seasoning:
- ¼ tsp salt
- 1/8 tsp ground black pepper

Directions:

1. Switch on a mini waffle maker and let it preheat for 5 minutes.
2. Meanwhile, take a medium bowl, place all the ingredients in it, reserving 2 eggs and then mix by using an immersion blender until smooth.
3. Spoon the batter evenly into the waffle maker, shut with lid, and let it cook for 3 to 4 minutes until firm and golden brown.
4. Meanwhile, prepare poached eggs, and for this, take a medium bowl half full with water, place it over medium heat and bring it to a boil.
5. Then crack an egg in a ramekin, carefully pour it into the boiling water and cook for 3 minutes.
6. Transfer egg to a plate lined with paper towels using a slotted spoon and repeat with the other egg.
7. Top chaffles with poached eggs, season with salt and black pepper, and then serve.

Nutrition : 265 Calories; 18.5 g Fats; 17.6 g Protein; 3.4 g Net Carb; 6 g Fiber;

Chaffle with Scrambled Eggs

Preparation Time: 5 minutes

Cooking Time: 10 minutes;

Servings: 2

Ingredients

- 2 tsp coconut flour
- ½ cup shredded cheddar cheese, full-fat
- 3 eggs
- 1-ounce butter, unsalted
- Seasoning:
- ¼ tsp salt
- 1/8 tsp ground black pepper
- 1/8 tsp dried oregano

Directions:

1. Switch on a mini waffle maker and let it preheat for 5 minutes.

2. Meanwhile, take a medium bowl, place all the ingredients in it, reserving 2 eggs and then mix by using an immersion blender until smooth.

3. Spoon the batter evenly into the waffle maker, shut with lid, and let it cook for 3 to 4 minutes until firm and golden brown.

4. Meanwhile, prepare scrambled eggs and for this, take a medium bowl, crack the eggs in it and whisk them with a fork until frothy, and then season with salt and black pepper.

5. Take a medium skillet pan, place it over medium heat, add butter and when it melts, pour in eggs and cook for 2 minutes until creamy, stirring continuously.

6. Top chaffles with scrambled eggs, sprinkle with oregano, and then serve.

Nutrition : 265 Calories; 18.5 g Fats; 17.6 g Protein; 3.4 g Net Carb; 6 g Fiber;

Sheet Pan Eggs with Mushrooms and Spinach

Preparation Time: 5 minutes

Cooking Time: 12 minutes;

Servings: 2

Ingredients

- 2 eggs
- tsp chopped jalapeno pepper
- 1 tbsp. chopped mushrooms
- 1 tbsp. chopped spinach
- 1 tbsp. chopped chard

Seasoning:

- 1/3 tsp salt
- 1/4 tsp ground black pepper

Directions:

1. Turn on the oven, then set it to 350 degrees F and let it preheat.
2. Take a medium bowl, crack eggs in it, add salt and black pepper, then add all the vegetables and stir until combined.
3. Take a medium sheet ball or rimmed baking sheet, grease it with oil, pour prepared egg batter on it, and then bake for 10 to 12 minutes until done.
4. Cut egg into two squares and then serve.

Nutrition : 165 Calories; 10.7 g Fats; 14 g Protein; 1.5 g Net Carb; 0.5 g Fiber;

Sandwich

Preparation Time*: 10 minutes*
Cooking Time*: 15 minutes;*
Servings*: 2*

Ingredients

- 2 slices of ham
- 4 eggs
- tsp tabasco sauce
- tbsp. butter, unsalted
- tsp grated mozzarella cheese
- Seasoning:
- ¼ tsp salt
- 1/8 tsp ground black pepper

Directions:

1. Take a frying pan, place it over medium heat, add butter and when it melt, crack an egg in it and fry for 2 to 3 minutes until cooked to desired level.
2. Transfer fried egg to a plate, fry remaining eggs in the same manner and when done, season eggs with salt and black pepper.
3. Prepare the sandwich and for this, use a fried egg as a base for sandwich, then top with a ham slice, sprinkle with a tsp of ham and cover with another fried egg.
4. Place egg into the pan, return it over low heat and let it cook until cheese melts.
5. Prepare another sandwich in the same manner and then serve.

Nutrition : 180 Calories; 15 g Fats; 10 g Protein; 1 g Net Carb; 0 g Fiber;

Scrambled Eggs with Basil and Butter

Preparation Time: 5 minutes
Cooking Time: 5 minutes;
Servings: 2

Ingredients

- tbsp. chopped basil leaves
- tbsp. butter, unsalted
- tbsp. grated cheddar cheese
- 2 eggs
- 2 tbsp. whipping cream
- Seasoning:
- 1/8 tsp salt
- 1/8 tsp ground black pepper

Directions:

1. Take a medium bowl, crack eggs in it, add salt, black pepper, cheese and cream and whisk until combined.
2. Take a medium pan, place it over low heat, add butter and when it melts, pour in the egg mixture and cook for 2 to 3 minutes until eggs have scrambled to the desired level.
3. When done, distribute scrambled eggs between two plates, top with basil leaves and then serve.

Nutrition : 320 Calories; 29 g Fats; 13 g Protein; 1.5 g Net Carb; 0 g Fiber;

Bacon, and Eggs

Preparation Time: 5 minutes

Cooking Time: 10 minutes;

Servings: 2

Ingredients

- 2 eggs
- 4 slices of turkey bacon
- ¼ tsp salt
- ¼ tsp ground black pepper

Directions:

1. Take a skillet pan, place it over medium heat, add bacon slices, and cook for 5 minutes until crispy.
2. Transfer bacon slices to a plate and set aside until required, reserving the fat in the pan.
3. Cook the egg in the pan one at a time, and for this, crack an egg in the pan and cook for 2 to 3 minutes or more until the egg has cooked to desire level.
4. Transfer egg to a plate and cook the other egg in the same manner.
5. Season eggs with salt and black pepper and then serve with cooked bacon.

Nutrition : 136 Calories; 11 g Fats; 7.5 g Protein; 1 g Net Carb; 0 g Fiber

Boiled Eggs

Preparation Time: 5 minutes
Cooking Time: 10 minutes;
Servings: 2

Ingredients

- 2 eggs
- ½ of a medium avocado

Seasoning:

- ¼ tsp salt
- ¼ tsp ground black pepper

Directions:

1. Place a medium pot over medium heat, fill it half full with water and bring it to boil.
2. Then carefully place the eggs in the boiling water and boil the eggs for 5 minutes until soft-boiled, 8 minutes for medium-boiled, and 10 minutes for hard-boiled.
3. When eggs have boiled, transfer them to a bowl containing chilled water and let them rest for 5 minutes.
4. Then crack the eggs with a spoon and peel them.
5. Cut each egg into slices, season with salt and black pepper, and serve with diced avocado.

Nutrition : 112 Calories; 9.5 g Fats; 5.5 g Protein; 1 g Net Carb; 0 g Fiber;

Enjoy
your meal

Conclusion

Start with non-processed carbs like whole grain, beans, and fruits. Start slow and see how your body responds before resolving to add carbs one meal at a time.

The things to watch out for when coming off keto are weight gain, bloating, more energy, and feeling hungry. The weight gain is nothing to freak out over; perhaps, you might not even gain any. It all depends on your diet, how your body processes carbs, and, of course, water weight.

The length of your keto diet is a significant factor in how much weight you have lost, caused by the reduction of carbs. The bloating will occur because of the reintroduction of fibrous foods and your body getting used to digesting them again. The bloating van lasts for a few days to a few weeks. You will feel like you have more energy because carbs break down into glucose, the body's primary fuel source. You may also notice better brain function and the ability to work out more.

The ketogenic diet is the ultimate tool you can use to plan your future. Can you picture being more involved, more productive and efficient, and more relaxed and energetic? That future is possible for you, and it does not have to be a complicated process to achieve that vision. You can choose right now to be healthier and slimmer and more fulfilled tomorrow. It is possible with the ketogenic diet.

This is not a fancy diet that promises falsehoods of miracle weight loss. This diet is proven by years of science and research, which benefits your waistline and your heart, skin, brain, and organs. It does not just improve your physical health but your mental and emotional health as well. This diet improves your health holistically.

Keto diet provides long term health benefits compare to other diet plans. During keto diet near about 75 to 90 percent of calories comes from fats, an adequate number of calories 5 to 20 percent comes from proteins and 5 percent of calories from carb intake.

What began as a simple spark of curiosity ended on a high note: keto, a term you constantly read and heard about. Now you have all the knowledge in the world to lead a lifestyle that is truly worthy of your time, energy, and effort.

Whether you have met your weight loss goals, your life changes, or you simply want to eat whatever you want again. You cannot just suddenly start consuming carbs again for it will shock your system. Have an idea of what you want to allow back into your consumption slowly. Be familiar with portion sizes and stick to that amount of carbs for the first few times you eat post-keto.

Being 50 years old or more is not bad. It is how we handle ourselves in this age that matters. Most of us would have just moved on and dealt with things as they would have arrived. That is no longer the case. It is quite literally survival of the fittest.

Do not give up now as there will be quite a few days where you may think to yourself, "Why am I doing this?" and to answer that, simply focus on the goals you wish to achieve.

A good diet enriched with all the proper nutrients is our best shot of achieving an active metabolism and efficient lifestyle. Many people think that the Keto diet is simply for people interested in losing weight. You will find that it is quite the opposite. There are intense keto diets where only 5 percent of the diet comes from carbs, 20 percent is from protein, and 75 percent is from fat. But even a modified version of this which involves consciously choosing foods low in carbohydrate and high in healthy fats is good enough.

Lightning Source UK Ltd.
Milton Keynes UK
UKHW050918180321
380562UK00002B/64